FATTY LIVER PROTOCOL

REGAIN YOUR YOUTHFUL ENERGY, IMPROVE YOUR
SLEEP, AND LOSE STUBBORN FAT WHILE FIXING
YOUR FATTY LIVER WITH DIET AND EXERCISE

DR. J. MATTHEW DURHAM

CONTENTS

Introduction   5

1. Liver 101   11
2. Not That Bladder   19
3. What Exactly is a Fatty Liver?   27
4. How Do I Know if I Have a Fatty Liver?   40
5. How to Fix Your Fatty Liver Starting Now   53
6. The Fatty Liver Diet Protocol: Food Rules, Meal Plans, and Grocery Lists   82
7. Time Your Eating and Exercise to Heal Your Fatty Liver   104
8. Recipes for the Fatty Liver Diet Protocol   116
9. Fatty Liver Diet Protocol Checklist and Final Advice   157

References   173

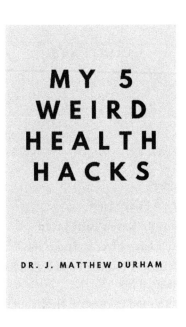

Included with the purchase of this book is my short guide, "My 5 Weird Health Hacks". These are also covered in this book but it is a great place to start if you are ready to jump right in on your road to health. Simply click the link below and let me know where to send it. Enjoy!

Get My Health Hacks - https://bit.ly/3zwivS6

INTRODUCTION

When Sarah walked into my office she had a familiar look of desperation in her eyes. She started talking and it was as if she could not pour her words out fast enough. I knew she was eager for help and as I listened to her reasons for coming to see me, I already had a sense of what her problem might be.

"Dr. Durham, I don't know what is wrong with me. Every day I struggle to get out of bed. I look at my to-do list and feel overwhelmed; I don't know how to get through even half of it. I'm just so tired and I have no energy to make it through the day. Between taking care of my children, their carpools, and their activities, I don't have any energy left to give to myself or my husband in the evenings.

I have also gained weight and nothing I do seems to

take off this belly bulge. I know I need to exercise, but the thought of the effort involved sends me reeling right now. I just want my life and my health back. I want to be able to play outside with my kids, go on bike rides with my family, and enjoy the little moments with them. And I want to be able to button my favorite jeans again.

I'm so frustrated and I want to know what I can do to get my health back. I just want to feel good again. Please help me."

As I dove deeper into Sarah's symptoms, her frustration was apparent and the bigger picture developed. I knew what was going wrong as we went through her concerns. Her fatigue, lack of energy, weight gain around her belly, hips, and thighs, sluggishness after eating high-carbohydrate meals, cravings for sweets, low libido, and constant abdominal bloating, all signaled that she was likely dealing with a fatty liver. She was not a drinker, so her sedentary lifestyle and poor food choices led me to believe that what she had was Non-Alcoholic Fatty Liver Disease (NAFLD).

That day, we began our journey of working together to heal her fatty liver and achieve the health she was looking for. I knew I could help her feel better about what she saw looking back at her in the mirror. My program would work for her because she was ready; she was ready to live her life to the fullest, ready to be active again with her family, and ready to achieve the vibrant health that she was longing for and missed so much.

I have been a practicing chiropractor, with a heavy emphasis on nutrition, in South Carolina since 1987. For the last 30 years I have been in the trenches, helping so many of my patients conquer the very issues that Sarah was struggling with as she lived with liver disease.

Sarah's symptoms were very typical of the many patients that I work with on a regular basis. Patients with fatty liver disease normally present with belly fat, a distended and bloated abdomen, constant fatigue, lack of energy, depression, regular heartburn, reflux, hemorrhoids, body odor, bad breath, itchy skin, and headaches. Further evaluation typically reveals high blood pressure, high cholesterol, low testosterone, and apnea.

NAFLD is the buildup of excess fat in the liver cells and is not caused by excessive alcohol consumption. NAFLD is becoming increasingly common around the world, and in the United States it is actually the most common form of chronic liver disease, affecting about one-third of the population. NAFLD is most commonly diagnosed in those who are obese or sedentary and those who eat a highly processed diet. Most are unaware that they even have a liver condition because they may not be big drinkers and their symptoms are vague, gradual, and non-specific in the early stages of liver disease.

The liver is the largest and hardest working solid internal organ in the body and is responsible for over 500 functions that include processing nutrients from food, making bile, removing toxins from the body, metabolizing drugs, breaking down fats, converting glucose into glycogen, and creating immune factors necessary to fight infections. When your liver is not functioning optimally, your body gives you signs to tell you that something is wrong. It is crucial that you do not ignore these hints, however subtle they may be, and make the necessary lifestyle changes to put you back on a path to health.

NAFLD is caused by a variety of lifestyle and environmental factors, such as diets high in refined carbohydrates and unhealthy fats, diets low in antioxidant-rich fruits and vegetables, prescription medications, recreational drug and alcohol use, exposure to environmental chemicals and toxins, and a propensity towards being overweight.

This is why I knew this book needed to be written. I knew I could help more people than just the patients that I can see in my own office. It was time to share my protocol with the many others that are suffering with NAFLD and may not know it, and show them that by making some necessary lifestyle changes you can rebuild your liver cells, reduce the damage, and feel better than you have in years.

If you are struggling with symptoms similar to Sarah's, then this book will give you true hope and the tools you need to change your life. I lay out a step-by-step nutrition plan that will give you back the energy, vitality, and excitement that you once had. At your fingertips you will have the blueprint to changing your life for good; just a little self-care for your liver can revitalize your health.

Today, Sarah is a vibrant picture of health. She is fitter and more energetic than she has been in ten years. She has lost over twenty pounds. When she came into my office recently, I could sense her joy and excitement as she told me how she finally feels sexy for her husband again; how she has been playing basketball every day with her son (and even beating him from time to time); how she took up mountain biking (and can beat her husband to the top now); and how, not only can she button her favorite pre-pregnancy jeans, but she now needs a belt to keep them up.

She finally understands how to properly care for her liver and her digestive health. She took the steps to heal and now knows that she will never again be that woman who walked into my office six months ago.

If you are ready, like Sarah was, to successfully conquer your own liver and digestive health issues and begin your journey towards thriving health, then this book will become your manual. It will teach you how to make healthy lifestyle changes to get your life, your weight, and your energy back for good.

1

LIVER 101

B efore we dive into the intricacies of the fatty liver, let us begin by taking a look at this incredible organ, its anatomy, and its functions to get a better understanding of what happens when it is working properly and what can go wrong when it is not.

WHAT IS THE LIVER?

The liver is the largest and most solid internal organ in the human body. The only organ that is considered to be both heavier and larger is the skin. The liver is also the largest gland in the human body.

Dark reddish-brown in colour and weighing around 3 lbs in adulthood, the liver is about the size of a football. This organ is a powerhouse and carries out over 500 roles in the human body.

It is vital to the body's metabolic functions and immune system and it is absolutely safe to say that without a functioning liver, a person cannot survive.

ANATOMY OF THE LIVER

The liver is located in the upper-right portion of the abdominal cavity. It is fairly triangular in shape and lies just beneath the diaphragm. A portion of the liver extends into the left-upper abdomen as well. It sits on top of the stomach, right kidney, and intestines. At any given time, the liver has a significant amount of blood flowing through it and holds about one pint, or 13%, of the body's blood supply. **(1)**

The liver receives its blood supply from two large blood vessels, the hepatic artery and the hepatic portal vein. The hepatic artery delivers oxygenated blood from the general circulation into the liver. This accounts for about 25% of the liver's blood flow. The hepatic portal vein delivers deoxygenated blood containing digested nutrients from the entire gastrointestinal tract, spleen, and pancreas into the liver. The hepatic portal vein supplies approximately 75% of the liver's blood flow. **(2)**

The blood received in the liver flows through the tissue to the hepatic cells where many metabolic functions take place. The blood drains out of the liver through the hepatic veins. The primary function of the hepatic veins is to deliver deoxygenated blood from the liver and other lower digestive organs (like the colon, small intestine, stomach, and pancreas) back to the heart through the inferior vena cava.

The liver consists of two main lobes: a larger right lobe and a smaller left lobe. The lobes are separated by the falciform ligament, a band of tissue that keeps the liver anchored to the diaphragm. The lobes are made up of eight segments that consist of lobules, the functional units of the liver. Each lobule is made up of millions of hepatic cells that are the basic metabolic cells of the liver.

These lobules are connected to a small duct that then connects with a larger duct to create a pathway to and from the common hepatic duct. The common hepatic duct transports the bile made by the liver cells to the gallbladder and duodenum (the first part of the small intestine) via the common bile duct.

KEY FUNCTIONS OF THE LIVER

As the largest organ in our body, our liver has three broad, essential tasks that are crucial to our bodies functioning properly: detoxification, synthesis, and storage.

Under these broad categories, the liver is actually responsible for more than 500 different functions. I will explain in depth how some of these functions are related to essential digestion and metabolism, detoxification, immunity, and the storage of nutrients within the body.

Digestion and Metabolism

Anything that is consumed through the mouth (food, medicine, supplements, alcohol, and even toxins) gets filtered by the liver after being digested by the stomach and the small intestines. The liver then processes nutrients so that they can be utilized by the rest of the body.

The cells of the liver (hepatocytes) produce a substance called bile, a mixture of water, bile salts, cholesterol, and bilirubin, that plays an important role in the digestive process. Bile is a greenish-brown, thick substance that passes through bile ducts to be stored in the gallbladder until a meal containing fat is eaten. The gallbladder is then signaled to release the bile into the first part of the small intestines (the duodenum). There the bile emulsifies the fat, making it easier for the body to digest and absorb it.

The liver is also able to convert simple sugars in the blood-stream into glycogen, which is better for storage. This makes the liver an energy center for the body because it helps control the fine balance of simple and complex sugar storages and controls the release of sugar stores when the body needs them for energy.

In addition to utilizing bile to help process fats and being able to convert simple sugars into glycogen, the liver also plays an important role in the digestion and processing of proteins by helping to create some of the essential building blocks that form protein, known as amino acids. Amino acids are essential for many vital chemical reactions. They are transported to the liver during digestion and most of the body's protein is synthesized here. If there is too much protein, amino acids can then be converted into fat and stored or made into glucose for energy.

The hepatocytes of the liver are responsible for many of the important metabolic jobs that support the cells of the body; almost all of the blood leaving the digestive system passes through the portal vein into the liver. This is what allows for the metabolizing of carbohydrates, fats, and proteins into material for the body to utilize.

Detoxification

When blood flows from the small intestines, spleen, and pancreas into the liver through the hepatic portal vein, the cells of the liver are on constant watch for any potentially toxic substances. If detected, they produce enzymes to metabolize these toxins, such as drugs and alcohol, into inactive metabolites that can then be removed through waste. The liver will also metabolize excess hormones that have been produced by the body and remove them from circulation through waste.

After these harmful substances have been broken down and made inactive, the remaining by-products are excreted into the bile to be sent to the intestines and eliminated as feces, or into the blood to be filtered by the kidneys and eliminated as urine.

Immunity

The liver plays an important role in immunity. It is designed to detect pathogens entering into the body through the intestines and to isolate and remove bacteria, viruses, or other infectious organisms that may be present in our food. This puts it at the forefront of our body's immune response.

The liver has the largest collection of phagocytic cells in the body. Phagocytes are cells that protect the body by ingesting harmful foreign particles, bacteria, and dead or dying cells. These phagocytes make the liver the body's frontline defense and allow it to mount a rapid and robust immune response to protect our bodies from foreign pathogens. So much blood passes through the hepatic portal system that the liver cells are able to clean a large volume of blood very quickly. Dynamic interactions between the large number of immune cells in the liver are key to maintaining balance and overall tissue health. **(3)**

Storage

The liver provides the storage for many essential nutrients, vitamins, and minerals that are obtained from digestion. Our liver is able to store vitamins A, D, E, and K, which are all fat-soluble vitamins, along with vitamin B-12, iron, and copper. By storing these essential nutrients, the liver is able to provide a constant supply to all of the tissues of the body. The reserves are released into the bloodstream from the liver when additional amounts of these important nutrients are needed.

In addition to the storage of these nutrients, the liver is also able to convert excess glucose into glycogen to store for later energy use. Glucose is the main source of energy for our cells. When the body needs additional fuel and it has not received it from current food sources, the body sends a signal for the stored glycogen to be broken down to release glucose back into the bloodstream where it can be used as fuel for the cells.

Other Important Functions of the Liver

While we have touched on the main functions of the liver, this incredible organ actually performs more than 500 functions, some of which scientists do not yet fully understand and are continually researching to learn more about.

Some additional responsibilities include:

- Regulating blood clotting
- Processing hemoglobin for the use of its iron content
- Producing certain proteins for blood plasma
- Converting poisonous ammonia into urea to be removed as waste
- Producing special proteins to help carry fats through the body
- Producing cholesterol which is used to make vitamin D.

All of these functions show that you cannot underestimate the importance of the liver and how essential it is to good health. It is a gatekeeper to any threats that your body may encounter and therefore needs to be cared for properly. Any signs of liver issues should be addressed immediately to put your body back on a path to optimal health.

Regeneration Abilities

In future chapters we will be discussing what can happen when your liver is not functioning optimally and what some of the signs and symptoms of poor liver function are. The effects of liver disease can have dire consequences on your health and body, and you need to be aware of the signs to look out for.

Fortunately for all of us, the liver has an incredible capacity for regeneration of dead or damaged tissues; it is capable of growing quickly to restore its normal size and function and can regenerate itself, even after large portions of it are removed.

This key function is the premise of this entire book. It is absolutely possible to put yourself on a better path to liver health because the liver is fully capable of healing itself. In the following pages you are going to uncover the secrets to a life filled with energy, vitality, and health. You are going to discover how you can lose your belly fat, get more restful sleep, and experience less daily pain. It will only take a few simple lifestyle changes, that you can gradually build upon, to make this shift happen and you will be well on your way to "You 2.0".

2

NOT THAT BLADDER

I cannot write a book about the fatty liver without addressing the key role that the gallbladder plays in your liver health. Unless you have had a gallstone, or had your gallbladder removed, you probably have not had a reason to think about this little organ. However, you will discover here that it is actually far more important than you realize and that it plays a key role in your digestion.

WHAT IS THE GALLBLADDER?

The gallbladder is a pear-shaped and hollow organ that sits beneath the liver on the right side of the abdomen. It stores and concentrates the bile made in the liver and then releases it into the digestive system as it is needed. It is part of the biliary tract, which includes the liver, gallbladder, and bile ducts; they all work together to make, store, and secrete bile. It is a muscular organ that contracts when the bile is needed, forcing the bile through the cystic duct into your small intestine to aid in digestion.

ANATOMY OF THE GALLBLADDER

In adults, the gallbladder measures approximately eight cm (3.1 in) in length and four cm (1.6 in) in diameter when fully distended. **(4)** It is located in front of the duodenum (the first section of the small intestines). While it is a small organ, it has the capacity to store approximately 30 to 50 cubic cm (cc) of bile at any given time. **(5)**

The gallbladder is divided into three sections: the neck (the area where the gallbladder tapers, becoming narrow as it joins the cystic duct); the body (the part of the gallbladder that begins to taper into the neck); and the fundus (the large rounded base where the bile juices are stored). The neck is what connects the cystic duct to the biliary tract. This then joins the common hepatic duct to become the common bile duct. When you hear about people getting gallstones, the place where the stones commonly get stuck is the neck of the gallbladder.

The gallbladder is attached to the digestive system by the biliary tree. The gallbladder and bile ducts make up what is called the biliary system (sometimes referred to as the biliary tract). Through this system, bile flows from the liver (where the liver cells make and secrete the bile) into the system of ducts that are located inside and outside the liver.

KEY FUNCTIONS OF THE GALLBLADDER

The gallbladder plays a key role in the digestive process. It is part of your biliary system, along with your liver and the associated ducts. This whole system is necessary for the production, storage, and secretion of bile.

The gallbladder acts as the storage centre and concentrator of the bile that is formed in the liver and then released when the body needs to digest fats. So while your liver manufactures bile, your gallbladder acts as the storage and release facility for it.

As mentioned in the previous chapter, bile is a thick, greenish substance that is made up of a mixture of water, bile salts, cholesterol, and bilirubin. It is necessary to convert the fats in food into fatty acids that can be absorbed by the intestines. Bile is essential for the complete digestion of fats, iron, calcium, and vitamins. The liver produces anywhere from 500 to 1,000 ml of bile per day, but the gallbladder can concentrate that bile tenfold and store up to 30 to 50 ml of the denser bile. **(6)**

Bile is also responsible for excreting unnecessary and unwanted chemicals and toxins from the body. It can eliminate excess copper, zinc, and mercury, along with other dangerous toxins. The toxins that are left after the liver detoxification process are secreted into the bile and then eliminated through the feces. Bile also serves as a way to help excrete bilirubin, which is the by-product of red blood cell breakdown, and carries excess cholesterol out of the body and into the intestines to also be eliminated through the feces.

It is also crucial in helping to stimulate bowel movements and prevent constipation. Because bile is made of fat, it provides a good lubricant for your stool. This one function alone makes it a very important part of the entire digestive process because fecal matter sitting in the colon for long periods of time can wreak havoc on your health, as we will discuss later.

COMMON GALLBLADDER PROBLEMS

If you are not eating the right foods or too much of the wrong ones, your gallbladder will eventually cease to work. You need to consume the right types of healthy monounsaturated and polyunsaturated fats in order for your gallbladder to function properly. The right types of foods (and specifically fats) to eat and those to avoid will be addressed in detail in later chapters as I begin to lay out the Fatty Liver Diet Protocol. You will find lists of what types of foods (and fats) to avoid and what types are ideal to enhance liver function and healing.

When you are consuming the right type of fats, your gallbladder will contract and release the right amount of bile to break down the fats and emulsify them so that your body can absorb them properly. Often, when you are eating a diet full of highly processed and hydrogenated fats, or when you are eating a diet that is too low in any type of fats, your gallbladder will not receive the messages that trigger it to release bile. When bile is not stimulated to be released, the bile can sit stagnant in the gallbladder and become too thick to be pushed out. This can lead to gallbladder complications such as the hardened stones of cholesterol or bile pigment that are more commonly known as gallstones.

When a gallstone blocks the flow of bile from the gallbladder to the small intestines, you may experience fever chills, weight loss, nausea, loss of appetite, itching, night sweats, severe pain in the upper abdomen, dark urine, and even greasy stools. Sometimes, you will experience no pain at all with gallstones, however, if a gallstone blocks one of the ducts in the biliary system, pain can occur. If left untreated, further complications can arise, sometimes resulting in the need for gallbladder removal.

Other common gallbladder complications include:

- Cholecystitis, which occurs when your gallbladder becomes inflamed and is usually due to a blockage caused by gallstones, tumors, infections, or even issues with blood circulation.

- Choledocholithiasis, which occurs when a gallstone blocks the common bile duct completely and bile begins to back-up into the liver. The gallstone can be removed from the duct using an endoscope, or the entire gallbladder may need to be removed to prevent a recurrence.

- Gallbladder polyps, which are growths that project into the gallbladder. These are typically noncancerous (benign) and do not usually cause symptoms. If symptoms do occur, then gallbladder removal may be necessary.

CAN YOU LIVE WITHOUT A GALLBLADDER?

Any of the infections or inflammation mentioned above can contribute to your doctor suggesting that your gallbladder needs to be removed. Cholecystectomy is the name for the surgical removal of the gallbladder. It happens to be one of the most common surgical procedures performed in the world. **(7)**

You can definitely survive without a gallbladder, however some lifestyle changes will be necessary to avoid any health or digestive problems. Because the gallbladder usually serves as storage for the bile produced by the liver, when you do not have a gallbladder, the liver has to release the bile directly into the small intestines. This means that bile may continually drip into your small intestines and irritate its lining. This can also lead to poor nutrient absorption. While the liver can release bile directly into your small intestines, allowing you to digest most foods, it may not be able to keep up if you eat a meal full of fatty and greasy food. You may end up feeling extremely gassy and bloated and suffer from diarrhea.

Some important dietary changes you can make if you do need to have your gallbladder removed:

- Limit the amount of fat in a single serving to no more than 3 grams.
- Try to spread your meals out to five or six smaller meals instead of 3 larger meals so that you do not overwhelm your digestive tract.
- Avoid fatty foods like chips, fried foods, and all seed oils such as vegetable oils or canola oil.
- Only eat foods such as bacon, sausage, and full-fat dairy in moderation.
- Include lean meats, such as lean cuts of beef, fish or skinless chicken, as your protein sources.
- Load up on vegetables, but only eat high-fiber vegetables, such as broccoli, cauliflower, and cabbage, in smaller doses so that your body is able to digest them properly.

My goal in writing this book is to help you identify potential problems with not only your liver, but your gallbladder too, both of which play a key role in the digestive process. Dietary intervention and lifestyle changes can help you preserve this organ. This book is an action plan which outlines the steps you need to take now to avoid or repair complications in the liver and gallbladder. Always remember that you are your own "study in progress", so as you follow these guidelines make note of what does work for you and what does not . Our goal is always a healthier, thinner, more energetic you!

3

WHAT EXACTLY IS A FATTY LIVER?

You are probably thinking: "Fatty liver? What does that even mean?" Fatty liver literally means that you have excess fat in your liver. You may have also heard it referred to as hepatic steatosis. Put simply, it occurs when the liver cells, known as hepatocytes, become so filled with fat that it affects their ability, and therefore the liver's ability, to function effectively.

Your liver is like a factory that never sleeps. As we discussed in earlier chapters, the liver is divided into three functioning parts: the processing plant, the distribution center, and the store-house. As your liver processes the blood that it receives from the body, it breaks down the nutrients from your food and distributes these vital nutrients back to the rest of your body so it can better absorb them. These nutrients help to make the blood plasma proteins and other key elements that are helpful in aiding digestion. The liver will hold on to any extra nutrients that you do not need to use right away and store them safely for future use. It also processes any toxins entering your body through your food and is able to eliminate them before they can harm you.

When your liver is functioning efficiently, it is the major fat burning organ in your body and is able to pump excessive fat within your body out through the bile and excrete it as feces. While a healthy liver will help keep your weight under control, an unhealthy liver will cause fat to build up in your liver and in the rest of your body. Your liver itself will become swollen and full of toxic fat. This begins to block the pathways that blood normally flows along and makes it difficult for the blood to be cleansed properly. When this happens, the blood that is returning to the heart is full of unhealthy fats and toxins and can damage your heart, and immune system as well.

When your liver becomes overwhelmed with too many toxins and fatty cells over time, it ceases to be able to do its job. It cannot function properly and this causes a backup in the liver. It also means that your blood will not circulate properly, important nutrients cannot be delivered to other vital organs, and your body cannot detoxify naturally, so even more toxins will build up in your liver. This vicious cycle is the result of fatty liver disease and it needs to be addressed by crucial lifestyle changes to prevent even more serious, and potentially fatal, health complications from arising.

HOW DID I GET A FATTY LIVER?

There are two main types of fatty liver disease: Alcohol-Related Fatty Liver Disease (ALD) and Non-Alcohol Related Fatty Liver Disease (NAFLD).

Alcohol-Related Fatty Liver Disease (ALD)

Alcohol-related liver disease is caused by the heavy consumption of alcohol. The liver breaks down alcohol, therefore, the more alcohol you consume, the more the liver needs to process, and the more damage is caused. The good news is that fatty liver disease related to alcohol consumption is preventable. And if you do have it, it can improve once you stop drinking.

If you do not stop drinking, however, serious complications can arise. Some of these complications include: an enlarged liver, which can cause pain and discomfort; alcoholic hepatitis, which is swelling in the liver and can cause jaundice, nausea, vomiting, fevers, and pain; and alcoholic cirrhosis, which is a buildup of scar tissue in your liver and can lead to liver failure if left untreated.

In addition to the above complications, about 30% of people with alcohol-induced liver disease have the hepatitis C virus and about 50% of them develop gallstones as well. People with alcohol-induced liver disease are also at greater risk of cancer of the liver, kidney problems, intestinal bleeding, fluid in the belly, confusion, and severe infections. **(8)**

While this book is focused on the healing of non-alcohol related complications with the liver, it is important to address how to repair alcohol-related liver damage as well. The goal in treatment is to restore normal function to the liver. The first step to making this happen is actually fairly simple. You must stop drinking alcohol completely. Oftentimes, this may involve treatment programs to help guide and support you. Dietary changes that will be addressed later in this book can also be very helpful for alcohol-related liver damage. If you believe that you have liver damage related to alcohol consumption, make sure to follow the plan that is laid out in this book to put yourself on the pathway to healing.

If the liver damage is severe enough, more serious treatment measures may be necessary. But no improvements or healing can begin unless an alcohol detox occurs first.

Non-Alcohol Related Fatty Liver Disease (NAFLD)

Non-Alcohol Related Fatty Liver Disease (NAFLD) refers to the accumulation of excess fat in the liver in people who drink little to no alcohol. The fat accumulates in the liver cells and begins to cause liver inflammation that can lead to different degrees of scarring and damage. NAFLD is a very common disorder and may affect as many as one in three to one in five adults, and around one in ten children, in the United States.

When NAFLD is left untreated it can lead to more serious conditions such as Non-Alcoholic Steatohepatitis (NASH). NASH is a serious condition that causes severe scarring of the liver and cirrhosis. Cirrhosis occurs when the liver cells are gradually replaced by scar tissue because of the damage done by the inflammation and fat accumulation. It is not uncommon to need a liver transplant once advanced cirrhosis occurs. The scar tissue impairs the liver's ability to function properly and repair itself.

WHAT CAUSES NAFLD?

The main focus of this book is to identify the causes of NAFLD and address the ways that you can actually heal and repair the damage in order to put your health back on track for good. There are several main causes of NAFLD that we are aware of.

Nutritional Deficiencies

Nutrition has a huge impact on the health of the liver. Those whose diets are high in refined carbohydrates and unhealthy fats, and low in antioxidant and plant foods, are at a much higher risk of NAFLD. Their dietary choices put them at risk of vitamin C, vitamin D, vitamin E, and selenium deficiencies, which are all necessary for liver health. Addressing these deficiencies and incorporating the proper sources of nutrition and micronutrients goes a long way to repairing liver damage and will be laid out in detail in later chapters.

Obesity, Type 2 Diabetes, and Insulin Resistance

One of the most common conditions thought to be a cause of fatty infiltration of the liver is obesity. It is believed that two thirds of obese adults and half of obese children may, in fact, have a fatty liver. About 20% of those who are obese may suffer from the more severe condition NASH. **(9)** But, in reality, it is not the obesity that causes NAFLD as much as NAFLD occurs as you are becoming obese.

The presence of type 2 diabetes and other metabolic conditions associated with obesity, including insulin resistance, are known risk factors for the development of fatty liver.

Insulin is a hormone secreted by the pancreas and its main function is to regulate the amount of nutrients, particularly glucose, fats, and proteins, circulating in your bloodstream. While insulin is usually recognized for its role in blood sugar management, it also greatly affects fat and protein metabolism as well.

Fat cells can only hold a certain amount of fat. When maximum capacity is reached, insulin will keep trying to put fat into the cells but they will refuse to accept it. While your pancreas continues to release insulin to attempt to lower blood sugar levels, your cells stop responding to this signal. This results in a rise of both blood sugar and insulin levels in your blood. This increase in production by the pancreas begins to tax this organ over time and it will eventually lead to a decreased amount of insulin being produced. When this occurs, your blood sugar will begin to exceed the safe threshold level and this causes type 2 diabetes.

One of the main factors that can contribute to insulin resistance is believed to be an increased level of carbohydrates in your diet. When you eat a meal containing a large amount of refined carbohydrates, the amount of sugar in your bloodstream increases. This signals the pancreas to release insulin into your blood, which then signals your cells to pick up the sugar from your blood in order to reduce blood sugar levels. When cells stop responding to insulin correctly and are unable to absorb any more glucose from the blood, insulin resistance occurs.

When the cells are unable to hold any more fat, the excess fat ends up being stored in and around all of your internal organs, including your liver cells. Once this occurs, you officially have a fatty liver.

Many researchers now believe that metabolic syndrome – the cluster of disorders that increase the risk of diabetes, heart disease, and stroke – plays an important role in the development of fatty liver.

Signs and symptoms of metabolic syndrome include:

- Obesity, particularly around the waist (abdominal obesity)
- High blood pressure (hypertension)
- One or more abnormal cholesterol levels — high levels of triglycerides, a type of blood fat, or low levels of high-density lipoprotein (HDL) cholesterol, the 'good' cholesterol
- Resistance to insulin, a hormone that helps to regulate the amount of sugar in the blood.

Of these, insulin resistance is the most important trigger relative to a fatty liver and is directly caused by the overconsumption of refined carbohydrates and, to a lesser degree, unhealthy fats.

Prescribed medications

Any substance that you take in by mouth, including all medications, are filtered through the liver. Typically this is a seamless and effective process. However, some medications can cause harm to the liver. Sometimes this harm occurs because the liver is already under stress and inflammation from other causes, making it more susceptible to damage from certain medications.

Some of the more common medications that can cause damage to the liver include:

- Pain relievers and fever reducers such as acetaminophen, ibuprofen, naproxen, and aspirin
- Cholesterol lowering medications commonly known as "statins"
- Tamoxifen, a non-steroidal antiestrogen used in the treatment and prevention of breast cancer
- Immuno-suppressants and analgesics
- Other classes of drugs including methotrexate, griseofulvin, steroids, valproate, and amiodarone. **(10)**

Recreational Drugs

Drugs taken for purely recreational use, including alcohol, narcotics (such as heroin, morphine, codeine, and hydrocodone), and amphetamines (such as methamphetamines), can cause severe liver damage, especially when taken in large doses.

Vitamin and Herbal Supplements

While I would argue that it is pretty rare, vitamins and supplements can also contribute to liver damage. You often hear how important it is to make sure you are getting enough vitamins and nutrients, but not all vitamin supplements are created equally and some can build up in the liver and actually cause damage.

Fat-soluble vitamins, including vitamins A, D, E, and K, are stored in the liver and fatty tissues of the body. While water-soluble vitamins, like vitamin C, can be removed quickly through the body, fat-soluble vitamins can accumulate in the liver and cause health problems if consumed in excess.

Too much vitamin A, for instance, taken over time can cause damage to the liver. Vitamin A-induced liver disease includes mild, but reversible, elevation in liver enzymes, hepatitis, and even liver failure. Some of the symptoms of vitamin A toxicity include bone and muscle aches, fatigue, headaches, and orange discoloration of the skin. Certain B vitamins can also cause liver damage if you consume them in excess; specifically, vitamin B-3 (also called niacin) taken regularly in high doses above 1000 mg.

Taking vitamins in moderation and not in high doses is the key to avoiding a toxic buildup in your liver.

Supplements and herbs can also cause liver toxicity because they are not regulated as carefully as other vitamins and medications. They can be sold with little to no testing in regards to safety or effectiveness; they have a higher chance of causing damage to the liver, especially if they have not been evaluated for impurities or toxins.

Some herbs that have been known to have negative effects on the liver include ma huang, skullcap, comfrey tea, and chaparral. Supplements being marketed for weight loss have also been known to cause significant damage to the liver as well.

In thirty-four years of practice I cannot recall a single case of "hypervitaminosis" or someone suffering from taking too many vitamins, but I have seen hundreds of patients that needed to add more vitamins or supplements to their diet.

Get your vitamins and supplements from a reputable source that knows how to set you up on a plan with proper doses. Most vitamins are made to be extremely safe at the recommended dosage. However, when you are dealing with a potentially life threatening condition such as NAFLD, do yourself a favor and get some help. This book is here to give you a plan to follow but it still would not be a bad idea to have a knowledgeable professional helping you along the way.

Environmental Toxins

The liver is responsible for cleaning toxins from the blood, therefore, overexposure to toxins can be harmful.

We are exposed to over 80,000 toxic chemicals in our environment on a regular basis. Once these toxins enter your bloodstream, your liver has to work especially hard to catch them and then effectively remove them from your body.

Exposure to these chemicals occurs through indoor air, outdoor air, drinking water, and food sources on a regular basis. Pesticides, fertilizers, and endocrine disruptors, such as BPA, TBR, and PFOA, seep into our food and water supply and are some of the biggest attacks on the health of the liver.

Plastics are known to release pseudo-estrogens. This is why you should never microwave food in a plastic container or wrapped in plastic wrap.

These toxins build up in the tissue of the liver over time, leading to increasing levels of damage. It becomes increasingly difficult to completely avoid them because these hidden toxins are everywhere.

Gut Dysbiosis

The microorganisms in the gut play a large role in the health of your liver as well. When you have too much of the wrong bacteria in your intestines, inflammation in your gut can occur. This inflammation in the lining of your intestines can lead to what is known as a "leaky gut". This then allows larger molecules to leak into the bloodstream that would not normally be allowed through the intestinal wall. These molecules often include unwanted toxins and other bacteria. The portal vein is a direct route from the gastrointestinal tract straight to the liver; this sends by-products of the gut bacteria into the liver where they can also contribute to fatty liver. The liver becomes exposed to bacterial endotoxins, such as lipopolysaccharide (LPS), that trigger an inflammatory reaction.

WHAT NEXT?

I have already said this, but it cannot be emphasized enough: the liver is *the* master detoxing organ of your body. So, if you are exposed to toxins in your everyday environment, through what you eat, what you wear on your skin, or what you drink or breathe in, the liver is exposed as well. When the liver becomes overloaded with these toxins, it is unable to work efficiently and can become bogged down with excess fat.

When the hardest-working organ of the body is not working properly, it may not be able to detoxify the blood efficiently enough and it may not be able to digest fats, break down hormones, or store the essential vitamins and minerals that are necessary for optimal health. As you will see in the next chapter, over time this can lead to symptoms that can progress in severity, signalling to us that it is time to make some serious lifestyle changes to reclaim our health and vitality.

4

HOW DO I KNOW IF I HAVE A FATTY LIVER?

WHAT IF I HAVE NO SERIOUS SYMPTOMS?

There are often very few symptoms in the early stages of NAFLD. The symptoms can be subtle and not immediately or easily attributed to a fatty liver. The majority of people with this type of liver damage may even have normal examination results in the earliest stages of the disease.

Even if you are not showing serious symptoms related to liver damage, you can still be experiencing dangerous health problems due to fat accumulation and inflammation in the body that can lead to damage and scarring in the liver. You are more at risk of liver disease if you have type 2 diabetes, obesity, hypertension, or high triglyceride levels in the blood. If you have any of these conditions you would most likely benefit from the lifestyle plan set out in this book. Not only will you be enhancing the health of your liver, you may also find that you lose weight and get your blood sugar and cholesterol levels back under control as well.

Some Symptoms to Watch Out For

One notable symptom, in both early and later stages of fatty liver disease, is upper-right abdominal pain. It sometimes begins as an inconsistent, dull ache or fullness, but as liver disease progresses, this pain can become more severe. You may also notice that you have stubborn weight gain around your abdomen that does not disappear no matter what you do, what you eat, or how much you exercise. But exercising will become increasingly difficult as a result of the fatigue that is associated with fatty liver disease. This fatigue might increase gradually until you find that you are struggling just to get through the day. Read on. You can get your energy back!

Many symptoms will initially seem vague and not obviously related to liver health when you are evaluating how you feel on a day-to-day basis. If you do have symptoms, they may include:

- Fatigue
- Jaundice
- Weight loss
- Loss of appetite
- Nausea
- Vomiting
- Confusion

- Trouble concentrating
- Pain in the center or upper-right part of the belly
- Enlarged liver
- Bloating and gas
- Constipation
- Pale or dark tar-colored stool
- Dry and dark patches on the neck and under the arms
- Swelling in the legs and ankles
- Weakness
- Excessive sweating
- Bruising easily
- Dark urine.

These symptoms will increase in severity as the disease progresses. The bad news is that once your symptoms have advanced, you are in the latter and far more dangerous stages of liver disease. Once the disease reaches this point, addressing, repairing, and healing the damage becomes far more difficult without medical intervention.

That is why the information in this book is so important. You have the ability, all by yourself, to stop the damage. You can change the entire trajectory of your health, starting today, if you are willing to make some important lifestyle changes. You will be amazed at the dramatic improvement in your health, your energy, your weight, and your attitude towards life once you start to follow the plan set out in this book.

If you are reading this book, then you most likely already suspect that you have some degree of damage to your liver and are probably experiencing some of the symptoms we have discussed so far. Getting tested early and understanding the severity of your disease is the most important factor in treating the condition. There are a number of tests that are available for this.

HOW IS FATTY LIVER DIAGNOSED?

Symptoms are vague when liver disease is still in the early stages; you may not even realize that you have an issue unless you have some routine testing done for another reason. Through that testing, it may be brought to your attention that you have abnormal blood markers or an enlarged liver. This may be your first indication of any trouble brewing in your liver.

There are several tests used to diagnose liver damage and fatty liver disease, either intentionally or unintentionally.

The "At Home Test"

I would describe this test as a screening to see if it is likely that you have a fatty liver rather than an actual test, but it is very useful as an indicator. You will need a tape measure for this screening. While standing, take three slow deep breaths and exhale fully. At the end of the third breath, while relaxed, measure the circumference of your waist at a point between your belly button and your pelvic (hip) bones on your sides. This measurement should be less than half of your height. If it is more than half of your height, there is a very good chance that you have a fatty liver.

A Physical Exam

Hepatomegaly, or an abnormal enlargement of the liver, is one of very few physical indications that you may have NAFLD. When the liver is larger than normal, this points to fatty accumulation and inflammation. This can be more difficult to assess in overweight or obese individuals where it is easily missed, so it is not a reliable form of detection.

It is possible that during a surgical procedure that is unrelated to a liver assessment, the doctor may recognize that your liver appears larger, more discolored, or differently textured than is deemed normal. All of these are also indicators of liver disease and should prompt immediate further testing and investigation.

There are not many obvious physical abnormalities that are easily detected during a physical exam, therefore, this is not a primary source of diagnosis for a fatty liver.

Blood Tests

A blood test can assess how well the liver is functioning. One of the most common blood tests determines the level of certain liver enzymes (proteins) present in the blood. In a healthy, functioning liver, the enzymes should mostly be contained within the cells of the liver so that the level of enzymes in the blood remains relatively low. However, if the liver is not working properly, these enzymes will spill over into the bloodstream. The enzymes that are the best indicator of how well the liver is functioning are the aminotransferases. These include the aspartate aminotransferase (AST) and alanine aminotransferase (ALT). When either of these numbers are elevated, it is a good indication that liver disease is occurring. These numbers can help the doctor assess the level of inflammation and damage, and additional blood tests may be ordered to find out if you have other health conditions that are increasing your liver enzyme levels.

Imaging

Routine imaging tests can show fatty deposits in your liver. There are several common types of imaging.

Ultrasound

An ultrasound uses a device called a transducer that bounces sound waves off of your organs to create an image of their structure. It is used to look at the size, shape, texture, and blood supply to the liver. If the liver appears very bright in an ultrasound image, this is indicative of fatty deposits in the liver. Cirrhosis can also cause a bright appearance of the liver tissue.

Computed Tomography (CT)

A CT scan uses a combination of both x-rays and computer technology to create an image of your liver. If the liver appears to have a lower density than other organs, this most likely indicates the presence of a fatty liver.

Magnetic Resonance Imaging (MRI)

An MRI scan uses radio waves and magnets, without using x-rays, to produce a detailed image of the organs and surrounding soft tissues. This type of imaging has the greatest sensitivity for diagnosing NAFLD, but does not do a good job of distinguishing the level of severity of the fatty liver.

Elastography

An elastography is a newer form of imaging that can help diagnose more advanced stages of liver disease, such as liver fibrosis. Some different types of elastography include: vibration-controlled transient elastography (which is a special type of ultrasound); shear wave elastography (a different form of ultrasound that determines liver stiffness); and magnetic resonance elastography (a special type of MRI to measure liver stiffness). (11)

Liver biopsy

A liver biopsy is really one of the only true means of detecting fatty liver disease. It involves taking a sample of the liver tissue through a fairly simple surgical procedure that involves ultrasound imaging and a needle. The sample can then be examined thoroughly under a microscope to identify if there are any signs of fatty liver disease, infection, inflammation, cancer, or scarring.

HOW SERIOUS IS FATTY LIVER DISEASE?

As I have discussed earlier, people with fatty liver disease often have no serious or extremely notable symptoms initially. In fact, it is often called a silent disease. The early symptoms do not cause a large disruption to daily living, so some people feel that it does not warrant any urgency in treatment. However, if left untreated, the disease can progress to a more serious and damaging condition called Non-Alcoholic Steatohepatitis (NASH). NASH can advance even further: total liver failure.

One of the biggest challenges with NASH is that most people who have it feel fine for a period of time or can easily ignore the early signs. They may not even know that they have a liver problem until the disease has reached the more advanced stages.

This is why it is crucial to understand how even the smallest symptoms can indicate fatty liver disease. Early diagnosis means that simple lifestyle and dietary changes can make a very big difference in the progression of the disease and in the health of your liver. If you wait too long to begin addressing these issues, serious complications arise and medical intervention will likely be necessary.

COMPLICATIONS WHEN NAFLD IS IGNORED

NASH

When NAFLD is left untreated, the damage can progress to steatosis with inflammation and hepatocyte necrosis (death of liver cells). This condition is commonly referred to as NASH. This occurs when your liver starts to lose function and begins to interfere with your ability to metabolize certain foods and medication. NASH is heavily influenced by daily lifestyle. Excessive calorie intake on a regular basis and a lack of physical activity are large contributors to the development of this disease and differ from fatty liver disease caused by alcohol or medication abuse.

Symptoms eventually progress in severity and become more attributable to liver disease as NASH becomes more advanced. Some signs to watch out for include muscle weakness; internal bleeding in the esophagus, stomach, and intestines; a buildup of fluid in the body (particularly in the abdomen); severe yellowing of the skin and eyes; and eventually even liver failure.

The most definitive way to correctly diagnose NASH is with a liver biopsy. As mentioned before, this is the best way to truly identify what stage of liver disease is present even if it is slightly more invasive and more expensive than some other forms of testing.

Fibrosis

When liver disease has progressed to NASH, the inflammation in the liver cells can lead to scarring in the liver called fibrosis.

Inflammation is a persistent cycle when you have liver disease. As a result of the inflammation, your body is constantly trying to repair the damaged cells in the liver by continually depositing collagen. However, the signal that a healthy liver would give to stop depositing collagen is interrupted because of the inflammation, so it continues to deposit more collagen beyond what is needed. All of that extra collagen begins to stiffen around the liver tissue. This build up of collagen, and other proteins, causing scar tissue formation is called fibrosis. **(12)** The scar tissue and regenerative nodules that are the result of the inflammation and fibrosis of NASH will replace healthy liver tissue and prevent the liver from functioning normally.

If detected early enough, fibrosis can be reversed through dietary and lifestyle changes and the underlying liver disease that caused the development of fibrosis can be cured or treated. If fibrosis is left untreated, however, it can lead to cirrhosis and liver cancer.

Cirrhosis

When the scarring on the liver becomes more severe and the damage is permanent, it is typically diagnosed as cirrhosis. While most people immediately think of cirrhosis as a result of alcohol consumption, it is actually just as common in NAFLD.

When liver damage is still in the stages of fibrosis, before it has advanced to cirrhosis, it is still reversible. However, there becomes a point where there is too much damage and the liver is beyond the point of being able to repair itself. As cirrhosis causes continued damage to the liver, excessive scar formation results in further loss of liver function and thus an increased risk of liver cancer and liver failure. At this point, medical intervention may be necessary in order to prevent liver failure. **(13)**

Liver Cancer

If cirrhosis advances far enough, one of the main complications is liver cancer. Liver cancer is the growth and spread of unhealthy cells in the liver. It is a leading cause of cancer-related deaths worldwide, but especially in the United States. **(14)** While other common cancers have seen an improvement in survival rates, liver cancer deaths continue to increase at an alarming rate.

It is rare to develop liver cancer without first having cirrhosis. This makes it especially important to receive regular testing and monitoring for liver cancer once you have been diagnosed with more advanced fibrosis or cirrhosis. The best survival chances occur when liver cancer is detected, diagnosed, and treated as early as possible.

Liver Failure

In advanced stages of liver disease, liver failure can occur. Liver failure happens when large portions of the liver are damaged beyond repair from severe scarring and inflammation. At this point, the liver cannot function any longer. The liver performs so many essential, life-sustaining functions, that when it can no longer perform these effectively, it becomes a life-threatening condition that typically requires urgent medical care.

Liver failure usually happens gradually over many years and is the final stage of successive liver diseases; a liver transplant may be a patient's only option. However, a transplant is a very risky surgical procedure associated with various complications.

HOW CAN FATTY LIVER DISEASE COMPLICATIONS BE PREVENTED?

At this point you should understand that the liver is one of the hardest working and most important organs in the body. To recap, some of the essential functions of the human liver include:

- Detoxification of blood from dangerous toxins and chemicals

- Production of important proteins
- Metabolizing and processing of essential nutrients and medications
- Processing of waste products of hemoglobin and other cells
- Storing of vitamins, fat, cholesterol, and bile
- Production and storing of glucose.

When the liver is not functioning normally, serious repercussions to your health can occur. In the following chapters I will outline a life-changing, step-by-step plan that will help stop liver damage in its tracks and put you on your own path to healing, repairing, and maintaining these crucial functions of your liver.

As part of this plan you will discover which foods to avoid, which foods to seek out, and how and when to include them; meal plans, grocery lists, and recipes; and even a checklist to keep you on the road to success. This plan is intended to be easy to follow and should become part of your daily lifestyle. By following this plan you will see big improvements in your energy, your weight, your mood, and your long-term health goals. You will feel better than you have done in years.

5

HOW TO FIX YOUR FATTY LIVER STARTING NOW

As I have discussed in the previous chapters, there are certain risk factors, in addition to genetics, that contribute to the development of fatty liver. Many of them are directly related to obesity, diabetes, high cholesterol, and other metabolic associated conditions.

Most of these risk factors are diet related and can be improved and fixed through some simple lifestyle and dietary changes. The liver is a rare organ that is self-healing and can actually repair itself from damage.

This gives you an incredible opportunity to take steps on your own to help your liver regenerate before the damage is too severe. It takes a proper understanding of what foods and lifestyle choices are causing harm to your liver and what changes you can make to put your liver back on track to health and healing.

The changes you make today and the results that you will see begin with you. Your dedication to your own health will ultimately determine the level of your success. With a few lifestyle changes and the step-by-step roadmap that I will lay out here, including meal plans, grocery lists, recipes, supplements, exercise suggestions, and a daily checklist, you will have every tool at your fingertips to be successful in your healing.

GETTING STARTED

It is very important to understand some of the conditions that predispose you to develop a fatty liver in the first place. The majority of these risk factors involve metabolic conditions, which means that you have the ability to control them.

In addition to genetics, some factors that will put you at risk of NAFLD include:

- Obesity, particularly when high levels of body fat accumulate around the abdominal area.
- High blood sugar or insulin resistance, which typically indicates pre-diabetes or type 2 diabetes. Once you have filled your fat cells to their limit from overeating carbohydrates and fats, insulin will begin storing fat in your liver cells causing fatty liver disease.

- High triglyceride levels; triglycerides transport and then store fatty acids within the plasma and blood cells. When your levels are high it can be a sign of NAFLD because the liver is the central organ for fatty acid metabolism.

- Sleep apnea; low nighttime oxygen levels can cause oxidative stress which is associated with the progression of NAFLD.

If you have been diagnosed with any of the metabolic-related conditions above, then you are at risk of NAFLD. The good news is that by making some positive lifestyle changes, you will not only see improvements in your fatty liver, but you will also see improvements in some of your other underlying health conditions as well.

FOODS TO AVOID WHEN HEALING YOUR FATTY LIVER

The liver removes toxins from the body's blood supply, regulates blood clotting, maintains healthy blood sugar levels, metabolizes and digests nutrients, and performs hundreds of other functions essential to a healthy human life. The liver needs to function optimally to be able to fulfil its essential roles. When you overindulge on foods that are not healthy for your liver, an accumulation of fat deposits build up in the cells of the liver. This makes it more difficult for the liver to function properly over time as it starts to get bogged down with this excess fat. This then leads to swelling and scarring of the liver. There are a variety of foods and drinks that are dangerous for your liver if they are consumed regularly.

Alcohol

While this is a book about non-alcoholic liver disease, when you are trying to heal NAFLD it is still wise to limit or even eliminate your alcohol consumption. Large amounts of alcohol will damage or destroy liver cells. When you combine alcohol with certain over-the-counter medications, the threat to your liver becomes even more dangerous. When your liver breaks down alcohol, the chemical reaction that results in this process damages your cells and leads to inflammation, cell death, and eventually to scarring and fibrosis. Alcohol can also block nutrient absorption which increases the toxic effects on the liver.

Sugary Drinks

Sodas, sports drinks, energy drinks, and fruit juice are full of sugar and artificial sweeteners that enter your body and contribute directly to fatty liver disease. Excess sugar consumption through drinks is easily overlooked and often not even thought of as a major source of sugar, but this hidden or silent sugar can lead to major weight gain and obesity. It is important to avoid and completely eliminate these sources of added sugar in your diet. Soda and sugary drinks are a deadly combination of both refined carbohydrates and sugar and are extremely detrimental to liver health.

Baked Goods and Refined Grains

Refined carbohydrates, like those found in most baked goods made with unbleached white flour, should definitely be removed from your diet when you are on a journey to healing your liver. Baked goods, white bread, pastas, even white rice, corn, and other "enriched" starchy foods, should be avoided because they are high in sugar and cause a spike in insulin production. Cakes, muffins, breads, and cookies can also lead to higher triglyceride levels in the body due to their fat content. It is essential to understand that highly refined grains convert into sugar once the body begins to process them and end up as fat in the liver.

Processed Foods

Any form of processed food can be dangerous to the liver. Processed fats are especially difficult for the liver to process. Limiting hydrogenated oils, such as vegetable oil and canola oil, and refined sugar is crucial when working to heal the liver. Avoiding all fast food and convenience foods is necessary on this trek to better health. Also limit sugar-laden yogurts, ice cream, and processed cheeses. All of these contain high concentrations of carbohydrates and the wrong kind of fats that will tax the liver as it works hard to digest and break these foods down. This overexertion leads to inflammation and fat buildup.

Foods such as canned soups and frozen meals, and snack foods such as chips, pretzels, candy, and chocolate should be eliminated from the diet as much as possible.

Foods High in The Wrong Fats

One of the odd things about fatty liver is that, for the most part, it is not caused by eating too much fat! It is the carbohydrates you have to watch out for! Protein and fat are very satiating which means they fill you up faster and keep you full for longer. Carbohydrates on the other hand are quickly converted to glucose and if not used right away will be converted to fat. Of course you can overeat fat but this is normally not a problem if you are just eating the fat that comes along with your protein and not eating the wrong kind of fat. It is important to switch to eating mostly healthy fats, but limiting your carbohydrate intake is going to be the core of your new diet program.

Fructose (the sugar in fruit, as well as high fructose corn syrup) is especially bad as it is almost always turned directly into fat and stored in the liver. While an occasional piece of whole fruit is acceptable, you definitely want to avoid fruit juice and fruit smoothies like you would alcohol while you are trying to heal your liver or avoid getting a fatty liver.

Foods that are fried in "seed oils" (corn oil, vegetable oil, and canola oil) are probably the worst thing you can eat from within the fat category, but particularly when you want to restore your liver's health. These are extremely high in bad fat and unnecessary calories. The liver is responsible for breaking down these fats and converting them into energy; these food items are high in the wrong kind of fats and are difficult to digest, so too much of these fatty foods will overwork the liver and result in the development of fatty liver disease.

Pesticides

The liver is the first line of defense against anything that enters the mouth and the bloodstream; it is important to consider that any types of chemicals that may be in your food will have to be metabolized and detoxified in the liver as well. Pesticides, used to grow non-organic foods, are considered to be extremely strong types of poisons. Sometimes they are so strong the liver is unable to remove them and these poisons can end up being stored in the liver. When these types of chemicals remain in the body, long-term health issues can arise and contribute to the inflammation associated with NAFLD. When working to restore liver health, it is imperative that you choose organic foods as often as possible to reduce your risk of exposure to these harmful chemicals.

SO WHAT *CAN* I EAT?

While it may seem like I just cut everything you enjoy eating out of your diet, you will be surprised at how many wonderfully delicious and nourishing foods you can fill up on to your heart's content, and that will actually help to cleanse and improve the health of your liver. It is important to reiterate that you do not get fat from eating fat and you do not get fatty liver from eating healthy fat; it is the carbohydrates that you need to watch out for. Below are some of the best foods for restoring optimal liver health.

Lean Protein

Lean proteins, such as beef, fish, seafood, pork, and chicken, are all rich in leucine, which is an essential amino acid that has been shown to help reduce fatty liver. Leucine improves glucose metabolism and reduces diet-induced insulin resistance. This directly affects the fat levels in the liver and can aid in reducing the effects of NAFLD.

Eggs

I consider eggs to be nature's multivitamin. They have gotten some bad press from time to time, but it never stands up to scrutiny. Simply put, eat as many eggs as you would like; at least four per day will get you the necessary choline and selenium you need to heal your liver.

Cruciferous Vegetables

Cruciferous vegetables, including Brussels sprouts, cauliflower, cabbage, broccoli, kale, collard greens, mustard greens, chard, bok choy, and watercress, support the liver's ability to detoxify the less-than-healthy foods that we consume. They act as a counterbalance to the harmful substances entering our body through our food, the air, and even our skincare products. This group of vegetables actually boosts the activity of detoxifying enzymes in our livers.

Coffee

Surprisingly, coffee (when taken black without creamers and sugar) has been shown to be especially effective in helping to improve fatty liver. It can reduce the gut's permeability so that the body absorbs less fat, and has therefore been recognized for its ability to help prevent the build up of fat in the liver. Coffee beans are rich in antioxidants so they can also help reduce inflammation in the liver.

Full Fat Dairy

Dairy products provide necessary nutrients that are not available in other food sources. Dairy only becomes a problem when you add in extra sugar, as with ice cream and most yogurts you see in stores. Of course, if you are lactose intolerant dairy is not your friend, but for those that tolerate dairy well, it is a great source of minerals such as calcium, magnesium, potassium, and even phosphorus. So feel free to enjoy some dairy.

Bright Purple and Red Berries

Berries, such as strawberries, blueberries, blackberries, and raspberries, are loaded with polyphenols and anthocyanins which supply antioxidants to reduce the damage caused by free radicals in the liver tissue and help to reduce inflammation and oxidative stress. They also help to improve immune cell response.

Garlic

Garlic is extremely rich in sulfur and selenium. Sulfur assists in activating liver enzymes, which help to flush out toxins. Selenium boosts natural antioxidant enzyme levels in the liver and helps to fight the damage caused by oxidative stress.

Artichokes

Artichokes are rich in the antioxidants cynarin and silymarin, which can help to reduce liver inflammation and lower fatty deposits. These antioxidants protect the liver from damage and promote the growth of new tissue. Artichokes can also increase the production of bile, which can help eliminate harmful toxins from the body. Artichokes are in the same plant family as milk thistle, which is an important herb used to improve liver health.

Water

More than half of the body is made up of water, therefore it plays a vital role in supporting proper liver function. Water is essential for liver detoxification and is important for cleansing the system of toxins and flushing waste from the body. It is also involved in stimulating bile production and helps to dissolve fats and soluble fiber. Staying hydrated keeps the blood thin, which makes it easier for the liver to filter. How much water should you be drinking? I get asked that question frequently.

The formula I like best is to take your weight, divide it in half, and drink that many ounces of water per day. So if you weigh 180 pounds, you would shoot for 90 ounces of water.

Healthy Fats

For many people, "vegetable oil" has become part of everyday life. Whether it is stir-frying a quick dinner, baking a cake, or deep frying french fries, almost every pantry in America holds a bottle of some sort of "vegetable oil". First of all, these are *not* vegetable oils; they are made from seeds by a process that uses dangerous chemicals. Secondly, they are Omega 6 oils; a prime example of the type of unhealthy fat we are trying to limit. To heal your fatty liver you will need to replace these unhealthy oils with healthy ones such as coconut oil, olive oil, avocado oil, or, dare I say it, butter!

Avocado

Avocados are an extremely important addition to your diet when you are working on improving your liver health. Avocados have a large amount of monounsaturated fat, antioxidants, and fiber, and they are one of the best natural sources for potassium. These are all especially helpful in improving liver function.

Fatty Fish

Fatty fish, like salmon, sardines, and mackerel, are rich in Omega 3 fatty acids. Omega 3 fatty acids have been shown to reduce liver fat and inflammation in people with NAFLD, so are a helpful addition to a diet regimen focused on reducing liver disease.

Flax and Chia Seeds

Flax and chia seeds are excellent plant sources of Omega 3 fatty acids, which, as mentioned previously, aid in reducing inflammation and fat in the liver.

Nuts

When eaten in small amounts, nuts can improve levels of liver enzymes because they are rich in Omega 3 fatty acids and antioxidants. Nuts that are particularly helpful for liver health include walnuts, almonds, pecans, and brazil nuts.

Probiotic Rich Foods

The gut and the liver are constantly communicating through the portal vein, therefore it is crucial that the good bacteria (probiotics) in the microbiome outnumber the bad bacteria. If this is not the case, then dysbiosis (an imbalance of gut bacteria) occurs which can trigger inflammation and a buildup of fat in the liver. It is very important to take steps to rebalance microbiomes so that beneficial bacteria can thrive and help the body to support optimal liver function. Probiotic rich foods, such as fermented vegetables, sauerkraut, kimchi, miso, kefir, and kombucha, are extremely helpful in shifting this balance of bacteria.

Organic Produce

It is crucial that you focus on organic produce grown without pesticides on a liver healing journey. It is important to remember that any types of chemicals present in your food will also have to be metabolized and detoxified in the liver. Eating organic vegetables whenever possible will help reduce the burden placed on your liver because there will be fewer harmful toxins for it to filter out.

IS THERE A SPECIFIC DIET I SHOULD FOLLOW?

There are many different diets that are helpful for a fatty liver. I am going to outline the diet approach that I believe is the most successful at helping people to heal their fatty liver. This approach blends together key aspects of a few different diets, particularly the ketogenic diet, a plant and protein based version of the Mediterranean diet, and the paleolithic diet. In my opinion, combining principles from all three of these dietary approaches allows for less restrictions and more options, and therefore an easier and more practical guideline to follow.

The main focuses of all three of these approaches are low-carbohydrate foods, quality proteins, nutrient-dense produce, and moderate amounts of healthy fats. There are endless possibilities for meals that will leave you feeling full and satisfied.

You will discover that there are so many more foods that you are able to eat in your quest to heal fatty liver than you would expect. In later chapters, I will lay out meal plans and recipes to show you exactly how many wonderful options you really have. You will be eating better than you have ever eaten in your life, all while healing your liver at the same time.

THE KETOGENIC (KETO) DIET

The ketogenic diet is a very low-carbohydrate, moderate-protein, high-fat diet. It involves drastically reducing carbohydrate intake and replacing it with fat. This reduction in carbohydrates puts your body into a fat-burning metabolic state called ketosis, where your body uses fat for fuel instead of carbohydrates. It also turns fat into ketones in the liver, which can supply energy to the brain.

When following a keto diet, the goal is to keep your carbohydrate intake below 50 g per day. This means you will not be consuming breads, grains, cereals, or even many higher glycemic fruits and vegetables. Carbohydrates are the main source of energy for the body; when this source is missing, the body will break fat down into ketones to use for fuel instead. These ketones can provide energy for the kidneys, muscles throughout the body, the heart, and the brain.

The main principles of a keto diet are:

- Eat mostly high quality fats (about 75% of calorie intake should come from fats)
- Consume moderate amounts of protein (about 20% of calorie intake)
- Consume minimal amounts of carbohydrates (no more than 50 g per day)
- Focus on grass-fed or free-range meats, wild-caught seafood (not farmed), grass-fed eggs, and organic leafy vegetables
- Only consume low-glycemic vegetables such as asparagus, avocado, broccoli, Brussels sprouts, cauliflower, cabbage, celery, chard, cucumbers, kale, lettuce, radish, spinach, summer squash, and zucchini
- Eat plenty of probiotic rich foods such as fermented vegetables, kefir, kimchi, kombucha, and sauerkraut
- Avoid all grains and beans
- Avoid fruits, except for berries (which are low-glycemic)
- Avoid starchy vegetables such as corn, carrots, parsnips, peas, potatoes, sweet potatoes, and yams
- Avoid all sources of sugar, including sweeteners.

Health Benefits of a Keto Diet

In addition to being used as a tool for weight loss, the keto diet has been shown to be beneficial for a variety of different health issues including:

- Reducing the risk and symptoms of conditions such as Alzheimer's and Parkinson's disease
- Improving memory function
- Reducing some symptoms of mental health disorders such as bipolar disorder
- Maintaining consistent blood sugar levels which helps to control or prevent type 2 diabetes and thus improves insulin resistance by lowering insulin levels to healthy ranges
- Reducing the frequency and severity of epileptic seizures in children.

THE PLANT AND PROTEIN-BASED MEDITERRANEAN DIET

When focusing on healing a fatty liver, one approach is a version of the Mediterranean diet that focuses on plant and protein based foods and that does not include a lot of grains. Prioritizing cruciferous vegetables, plenty of green leafy vegetables, beans, nuts, olive oil, herbs, spices, dairy, fish, lean meats, and poultry are principles essential to the healing of the fatty liver. This diet also focuses on a low-carbohydrate approach which is crucial to improving and eliminating insulin resistance, which plays a large role in NAFLD.

The main principles of this version of the Mediterranean Diet include:

- Consuming plenty of organic vegetables and some fruits, mostly berries
- Adding nuts, seeds, extra virgin olive oil, and coconut oil to your diet
- Eating plenty of fish, lean meats, poultry, full fat dairy, and grass-fed eggs
- Limiting or completely eliminating processed meats, refined carbohydrates and sugars, and processed and packaged foods.

The Mediterranean diet is based on the cuisine and cultures of the countries bordering the Mediterranean Sea, but focuses particularly on the foods common in Spain, Italy, Croatia, and Greece. While exact foods and combinations of these foods may vary in each of the countries, they all share some specific common features. Most importantly, each of these country's cuisines minimizes the use of processed foods and instead centers around fresh and local produce, seafood, legumes, lean meat and poultry, and olive oil.

The beautiful thing about the Mediterranean diet is that there is not one perfect or right way to follow the diet, as long as you focus on fresh, unprocessed ingredients and include antioxidant-rich plant foods and lean sources of meat, fish, and eggs. Meals in the Mediterranean diet emphasize a plant-based eating approach that is jam-packed with vegetables and healthy fats like olive oil and Omega 3 fatty acids from seafood, nuts, and seeds. The Fatty Liver Diet Protocol does eliminate sugary foods and allows for plenty of seafood, but not at the expense of red meat and full fat dairy; so while we will use some of the aspects of this diet we will not be following a strictly Mediterranean diet to reverse our fatty liver.

The Mediterranean approach is a way of life rather than simply a "diet", which is why I like to incorporate a few of the principles into my own fatty liver healing lifestyle. The benefit of this way of eating is that it does not completely eliminate entire food groups or restrict calorie intake like some diets do.

Health Benefits of the Mediterranean Diet

There are many important health benefits of a modified version of the Mediterranean diet. These benefits include improved liver and heart health, improved brain cognition, lowered risk of diabetes, increased motivation to exercise, and even cancer prevention.

This way of eating has been widely researched, and some of its principles have been shown to help in the reversal of NAFLD. (16) It has been a useful source of information to help formulate The Fatty Liver Diet Protocol.

THE PALEOLITHIC (PALEO) DIET

The paleolithic diet focuses on eating what our ancestors ate, before agriculture, animal farming, and processed foods were part of civilization. The premise is that our bodies function more effectively when fueled with nutrient-dense foods that can be hunted and gathered versus more modern foods like legume, grains, and dairy products.

A paleo approach is meant to be lower in carbohydrates and prioritizes foods that are lower on the glycemic index. The glycemic index categorizes foods containing carbohydrates based on how quickly or slowly they are broken down and how quickly or slowly they affect your blood sugar. By consuming foods which are broken down more slowly and cause a gradual rather than rapid rise in blood sugar levels, such as non-starchy vegetables, blood sugar levels can be managed more effectively and insulin sensitivity can improve.

Foods eliminated on this diet include grains, all dairy, all legumes, vegetable oils, hydrogenated oils, sugar and high-fructose corn syrup, processed foods, and artificial sweeteners. The focus is on removing processed and refined foods, and foods which have no nutritional value (empty calories), from your diet.

Encouraged foods include meat and poultry, liver, wild-caught seafood, pastured eggs, nuts (except peanuts), seeds, fruit, vegetables, sweet potatoes, yams, herbs, spices, coconut oil, avocado oil, and extra virgin olive oil. These nutrient-dense whole foods improve health by providing all of the nutrition that your body requires.

The main principles of the paleo diet include:

- Avoiding all grains, including rice, wheat, corn, sorghum, and oats
- Avoiding sugar in all forms; this includes all forms of sweeteners, such as cane and coconut sugar, maple syrup, corn syrup, agave nectar, honey, and artificial sweeteners
- Avoiding all hydrogenated fats
- Enjoying generous amounts of natural fats from avocados, animal fats, ghee, unrefined coconut oil, lard, olive oil, and nuts
- Avoiding all soy products
- Avoiding beans and other legumes (lentils, peanuts, kidney beans, black beans, soybeans)
- Eating only high-quality meat, preferably from organic, grass-fed (as opposed to grain-fed) animals, and avoiding meats treated with antibiotics and hormones
- Eating eggs from free-range chickens
- Eating poultry from free-range birds
- Eating wild fish and shellfish, rather than farm-raised seafood
- Enjoying fruit, but only in moderation: fruit is high in

a form of sugar called fructose which is particularly hard on the liver; berries are the fruit with the lowest sugar content and are most suitable for the paleo diet

- Enjoying lots of vegetables; however limiting sweet potatoes and eliminating regular potatoes
- Limiting dairy, except for butter and ghee
- Enjoying fermented and cultured foods like sauerkraut and kimchi for gut health
- Sipping bone broth
- Eating plenty of nuts including walnuts, macadamia nuts, pine nuts, almonds, and cashews.

Health Benefits of a Paleo Diet

One of the main health benefits of a paleo diet is that you are eliminating processed, packaged, and chemical- and preservative-laden foods. This approach is instead based on clean, high-quality foods with a focus on vegetables, plants, nuts, seeds, high-quality meats, and healthy oils. As a result, you are consuming nutrient-dense, anti-inflammatory foods that lower the risk of developing type 2 diabetes, heart disease, liver disease, and even dementia.

Another benefit of the paleo diet is that you will be primarily eating foods that are lower on the glycemic index, therefore you will be reducing the demand on the pancreas to produce insulin. This can drastically improve insulin resistance and help to avoid or reduce the symptoms of type 2 diabetes as well.

Calorie counting or restriction are not part of the paleo diet. It does not limit the amount of food you are eating, it only eliminates certain types of food. It is helpful to think of this approach as a new lifestyle rather than a restrictive "diet". You will not feel deprived or be forced to go hungry, so the chances of successful follow through are far higher.

A COMBINATION OF THESE PRINCIPLES: THE FATTY LIVER DIET PROTOCOL

All three of the diet approaches that I have discussed emphasize high-quality proteins and fats, nutrient-rich plants, and avoidance of carbohydrate-rich processed and sugary foods. The combination of these approaches forms the basis of The Fatty Liver Diet Protocol. This diet protocol will help to prevent NAFLD or combat it if it is already present.

As we have discussed, obesity and insulin resistance play a major role in the development of NAFLD and its progression towards NASH. To recap, insulin is a hormone secreted by the pancreas and its main function is to regulate the amount of nutrients, particularly glucose, fats, and proteins, circulating in your bloodstream. While insulin is usually recognized for its role in blood sugar management, it also greatly affects fat and protein metabolism as well. Insulin resistance occurs when we consume so many carbohydrates that there is nowhere to store excess glucose in the blood.

It is believed that two thirds of obese adults, and even as many as half of obese children, may have a fatty liver. About 20% of those who are obese suffer from the more severe condition NASH. **(9)** The link between NAFLD and type 2 diabetes is also very strong. Up to 70% of obese patients with type 2 diabetes have NAFLD. Therefore, the presence of type 2 diabetes, insulin resistance, and other metabolic conditions linked with obesity, are major risk factors associated with the development of fatty liver.

Following a diet protocol that focuses on nutrition to help repair your fatty liver, means that you will be able to target all of these associated metabolic conditions as well.

Potential Health Benefits

There are a variety of health benefits associated with The Fatty LIver Diet Protocol beyond healing your fatty liver.

Improved Heart Health

There has been a huge amount of research into the way that diet can help to improve heart health. This diet can reduce the likelihood and severity of heart disease by lowering the body's levels of "bad" cholesterol (LDL), and reduces the risk of other cardiovascular conditions, including heart attacks and strokes. **(17)**

Reduced Blood Pressure

Blood pressure is an important marker for many diseases and conditions, including heart disease and stroke. Maintaining a healthy blood pressure is a key component of healthy living. Following these principles of eating can reduce high blood pressure, thus reducing the likelihood of the serious associated health risks. **(18)**

Reduction in Inflammatory Bowel Diseases

This diet is devoid of inflammatory sugars, carbs, and seed oils, so it can help to reduce inflammation in the intestinal tract that typically causes digestive diseases. It will improve gut health as well.

Reduction in Cognitive Decline

Some studies now show that many, if not all, of the neurode-generative diseases of the brain, such as Alzheimers and Parkinsons, are rooted in a breakdown in the glucose metabolism pathway. Eating a low-carbohydrate, high-protein diet will require your body to use ketones for fuel. This bypasses the glucose metabolic pathway and can lead to an improvement in brain activity and a reduction in cognitive decline. This diet also encourages the consumption of low-glycemic berries which can directly support the brain by protecting it from oxidative stress and inflammation; they have been shown to help prevent depression and dementia-related diseases such as Alzheimer's disease.

Reduced Risk of Cancer

Studies show that adhering to a diet that is focused on nutrient-rich foods and that limits the intake of carbohydrates may also reduce the risk of colorectal, breast, and prostate cancer. This is due to the promotion of foods with high levels of anti-inflammatory and antioxidant nutrients. These nutrients protect against developing cancer and support recovery if cancer has already developed. **(19)**

SUPPLEMENTS FOR LIVER HEALTH

Please note: Before starting any vitamin or supplement regimen, it is very important to first consult your healthcare provider.

At this point you should understand that without a properly functioning liver, it is impossible to have a healthy working metabolism. You should get the majority of the nutrients that are essential for effective liver function from the food sources I have already discussed. However, it can be difficult to actually consume the necessary amounts of these nutrients, enough to encourage healing and fat and inflammation reduction, from food alone. Maintaining a healthy lifestyle with a nutrient-rich diet and exercise will naturally aid liver function, but additional supplements can enhance liver health and make great advances in repairing fatty liver damage. Below I will go through some of the supplements that can have the greatest positive effects on the health of the liver.

SEVEN IMPORTANT SUPPLEMENTS TO CONSIDER

Probiotics

It is very important to take steps to rebalance microbiomes so that beneficial bacteria can thrive and help the body support optimal liver function. Probiotic rich foods, such as fermented vegetables, sauerkraut, kimchi, miso, kefir, and kombucha, are extremely helpful in shifting this balance of bacteria. While food and drink sources of probiotics are ideal, they do not always provide enough good bacteria. A quality probiotic supplement which combines multiple bacteria strains is helpful in ensuring you are getting enough probiotics to keep your bacteria in balance and help repair and heal liver function.

Milk Thistle

Milk thistle is one of the most popular supplements for treating and repairing the liver thanks to its amazing seeds, which contain a flavonoid called silymarin. Milk thistle is an herb that has been extremely well researched for use in the treatment of liver disease and is thought to reduce damage to the liver caused by free radicals, which are produced when your liver metabolizes toxic substances.

The silymarin component in milk thistle is a powerful antioxidant that can help to optimize liver detoxification and liver function by acting as a guard against toxins and free radicals that may damage the liver. It can block these free radicals from entry into the liver cells and destroy the toxins that have already made their way into the cells. In addition, milk thistle can also increase the body's production of the powerful antioxidant glutathione, and help prevent the depletion of it in the liver, where the majority of it is stored.

Artichoke Leaf Extract

Artichokes support liver and digestive health by regulating blood sugar levels, helping with cholesterol metabolism, and potentially aiding in decreasing levels of fat in the liver. Artichokes are rich in phytochemicals such as phenolic compounds, flavonoids, and inulin (a prebiotic fiber). Phytochemicals like these act as antioxidants to protect against oxidative stress and damage.

Artichoke extract contains cynarin which promotes bile secretion; this is crucial for fat digestion and clearing dangerous toxins from the bloodstream. Cynarin promotes liver detoxification and protection, and it can encourage normal body mass index and limit complications from obesity. Like milk thistle, artichoke leaf extract also contains the flavonoid silymarin – the benefits of which are explained above. Artichoke leaf extract is a very important addition to a liver supplement program.

Ginger

Ginger supplementation can help reduce the risk of developing NAFLD or, if the disease has already developed, can aid in improving and repairing the damage already done. It reduces oxidative stress on the liver, decreases insulin resistance, and its anti-inflammatory properties reduce liver inflammation. Supplementing with ginger can also enhance the effectiveness of other lifestyle changes.

Vitamin E

Vitamin E is an extremely powerful antioxidant that can help reduce inflammation and fat content in the liver, improve fibrosis, and help decrease liver cell death. It can also potentially improve liver function by neutralizing free radicals, which prevents the progression of NAFLD to more severe forms of the disease.

Dandelion Root Extract

Dandelion root can lower inflammation levels in the liver, support the production of bile, and remove harmful toxins so that your liver does not have to work as hard during the detoxification process. It may reduce levels of excess fat stored in the liver and protect against oxidative stress in the liver tissue. These benefits all help to avoid or counter NAFLD.

Choline

Choline helps to clear the liver of cholesterol, which prevents NAFLD as well as a number of other diseases and conditions including heart disease and strokes. Choline is found in meat and eggs; if you are eating a higher-protein diet as described in this book, there is a good chance you will not need a choline supplement. Four eggs will give you all of the choline you need to heal your fatty liver over time. As well as choline, eggs contain many other beneficial nutrients including healthy fats, protein, and B vitamins; I consider them to be "nature's multivitamin" and I cannot recommend them enough. If you are allergic or intolerant to eggs, a choline supplement will be very beneficial.

6

THE FATTY LIVER DIET PROTOCOL: FOOD RULES, MEAL PLANS, AND GROCERY LISTS

In the following pages you will find meal plans, grocery lists, and nutritional guidance. If you are committed, these tools will allow you to adopt a lifestyle that will change the health of your liver for good.

A clean, fresh, and healthy diet – that is low in carbohydrates but high in quality fats, nutrient-dense produce, and lean proteins – is necessary to heal your fatty liver, boost your metabolism, and lose weight. The guidelines, strategies, and key rules that are outlined in the following pages will help you to follow the Fatty Liver Diet Protocol and assist you on your journey towards optimum health.

GUIDELINES FOR SUCCESS

1. Ditch the word "diet"

The "D" word *only* equates to short term success. Diet changes are necessary to address fatty liver disease, but instead of thinking of this as a diet, think of it as a new lifestyle. Lifelong changes deliver permanent results.

2. Ditch all grains

Store-bought breads, crackers, muffins, and snacks are usually filled with starchy carbohydrates that will spike insulin levels and add a layer of visceral fat around your middle. If you want to eat some form of baked goods, you can bake your own using high-fiber coconut flour or almond flour.

3. Begin a love affair with the perimeter of your grocery store

Vegetables, seafood, lean meats, poultry, nuts, and seeds are all found around the edges of most grocery stores and are incredible foods for healing a fatty liver.

4. Spice it up

While you are in the midst of the aforementioned love affair with the perimeter of your grocery store, do take a detour down the spice aisle. Getting creative with your spices and herbs can take a bland meal and turn it into a delicious family favorite.

5. Plan your meals out at the beginning of the week

Keep your meal plan and shopping list close and get everything you need at the beginning of the week so it is all on hand and ready to go.

6. Eliminate all packaged foods from your pantry

Eat *only* whole fresh foods and meals made with simple ingredients. As I often tell patients, the first step to better nutrition is learning to read labels. The second step is learning to eat mostly foods that do not have labels!

7. Focus on taking care of your gut...from the inside out

Prioritising gut health and taking care of your digestion will make a big contribution to healing your fatty liver. Probiotic rich foods and probiotic supplements are one way to go about this.

8. Keep meals simple

Keep your meal ingredients to a minimum. Focus on your protein and go from there. Create fresh and easy meals that only take minutes to throw together. This will keep you on track and stop you from falling off the wagon because meal preparation is getting "too hard" or because it takes "too long". Some of the simplest meals can taste and make you feel the best when all you are using are fresh wholesome ingredients. The recipes at the end of this book fall into that category. They will get you in and out of the kitchen fast and you will end up with an amazing meal.

9. Be realistic

We are faced with many temptations and time restraints every day. Setting goals is important but we should not set ourselves up for failure. Decide upon a goal that is challenging but doable. For example, aim to lose 2–5 lbs by a certain date. When you have met this first goal, set a new goal until you reach your ideal weight. These goals are more focused and achievable than simply setting out to lose 20 pounds. Of course, you should not limit your goals to weight loss alone; health and exercise goals are just as important.

10. Plan Ahead

Failing to plan is planning to fail. Try not to fly by the seat of your pants. Make grocery lists, plan what you will take to the office for lunch, know ahead of time what you can eat on those days you know you will not have time to spend in the kitchen, and pack healthy snacks for long days and outings. It can also be useful to prepare vegetables on the day you buy them so that they are ready to use for cooking; this will save time later. Planning will remove any opportunities for bad habits to sneak back in and will go a long way to maintaining and repairing health.

THE RULEBOOK

Three Key Rules

Every day, and no matter what, you must follow these three key rules.

1. Start each day with half of a lemon squeezed into 8–10 ounces of water

Make sure you drink the entire glass. Lemon water helps our bodies to flush out toxins and restore the liver. Lemon water can also help digestive health, weight loss, exercise performance, mental health, hydration, and the body's pH balance.

2. Drink water... and then drink more water... all day long

Water helps with energy levels, digestion, and hunger; it also has no calories. If you are eating increased calories, the last thing you want to do is add in high-calorie drinks like sodas, fruit juice, punches, and alcohol. If you are cutting out high-calorie foods, you do not want these drinks to undermine your efforts. Aim for 8–10 glasses of water per day.

3. Drink plenty of bone broth

You can buy fresh, organic, grass-fed bone broth from a variety of health food stores, or you can make your own using the recipe in this book (this is the most cost-effective method). Use this homemade miracle broth whenever broth is called for in a recipe. Bone broth can help reduce insulin levels, boost immunity, reduce inflammation in the gut, and aid in weight loss.

"No's" to Live By

- No alcohol
- No refined flour products; bread, bagels, crackers, cakes, wraps
- No protein or energy bars (these are usually just disguised candy bars)
- No desserts or candy; chocolate bars, ice cream, candy, cookies
- No deli meats or processed meats with nitrites or breading
- No artificially sweetened diet foods or beverages
- No pre-packaged microwave meals or snack foods
- No foods with artificial colors or flavors
- No soy or soybean oil, or any other "seed oil"
- No sugar or sweeteners
- No fruit or fruit juice (yes, you read that right; fruit is high in fructose and too much fructose is terrible for your liver when it is trying to heal).

Feed Your Body These Fat-Burning Foods

- Free-range, organic, and antibiotic-free poultry, beef, pork, bison, turkey, and pastured omega-rich eggs

- Wild salmon, trout, and sardines; canned is fine
- Unsalted and unsweetened nuts and seeds; limit each serving to a small handful
- Coconut oil, olive oil, fish oil, and Omega 3 EFA's (fatty acids).

Stick to These Beverages

- Filtered water with fresh lemon
- Green or white tea
- Sparkling seltzer; avoid varieties with artificial flavors
- Kombucha; be aware of the sugar content
- Bone broth.

Eat Only Low-Carbohydrate Berries and Vegetables

- Vegetables & leafy Greens; asparagus, broccoli, cauliflower, green beans, spinach, cucumber, celery, peppers, kale, chard, parsley, asparagus
- Organic mixed berries; frozen or fresh blueberries, strawberries, blackberries, and raspberries
- Find a full list at the end of this book.

Eat Only High-Quality Proteins

- Whole Omega 3 eggs (2–3 for snacks, 3–6 for meals)

- Grass-fed beef (eye of round, top round, and brisket), bison, and pork (tenderloin)
- Chicken and turkey; including chicken or turkey sausage and bacon rather than pork
- Seafood; white fish (cod), salmon, trout, light tuna, canned sardines, oysters, mussels
- Find a full list at the end of this book.

Eat Only High-Quality Fats

- Butter
- Olives, extra virgin olive oil, olive oil mayonnaise
- Coconut oil
- Avocados and natural guacamole
- Find a full list at the end of this book.

Sticking to the Rules

While these rules may seem overwhelming initially, you will soon find that they become an unconscious part of your everyday routine. The benefits to following these principles far outweigh the initial work involved.

1. There are endless meal options and combinations

There are so many whole, fresh foods to choose from that you will never get bored; you will not run out of meal ideas and you will not feel like you are eating the same things over and over.

2. It is not restrictive at all

While I would never recommend a vegan or vegetarian diet, the Fatty Liver Diet Protocol can incorporate dietary preferences, including vegetarian, vegan, gluten-free, and dairy-free. Anyone can find a way to thrive through these nutrient-dense whole foods and the huge variety of high-quality meat, seafood, eggs, vegetables, low-glycemic berries, nuts, and seeds that are available.

3. It will become a lifestyle, not a "diet"

These changes are simple to incorporate into your daily life and are easy to sustain in the long term. You do not need to cut calories; you just need to incorporate lean meats, eggs, antioxidant-rich plant produce, legumes, seeds, and seafood as often as possible and eliminate foods that are high in unhealthy fats. The ultimate goal is to create positive lifestyle and nutritional changes that will lead to long-term success.

It is quick and easy to see results in your health, fatty liver reduction, and weight loss when you are focused on these diet and lifestyle changes as part of every meal. Your body is going to function at its best when it is being nourished with good food. Instead of focusing on the things that you cannot eat, focus on the thousands of nourishing options that are available to you.

TWO WEEK MEAL PLAN AND GROCERY LIST

The meal plans that are laid out here will cover your first two weeks on the Fatty Liver Diet Protocol and will help you to get accustomed to this new way of cooking and eating. The meal plans include three meals plus snacks, so you should not feel hungry.

After the first two weeks, you can continue to use these meal plans as a guide by substituting in new meals. There are many additional recipes and lists of healthy foods at the end of this book to give you even more ideas and options as you continue on your nutritional journey. As long as you are following the rules in this book and eating only the recommended foods, you will begin to notice big improvements in your health, your energy levels, your weight, and the state of your liver.

Below I have outlined some tips for success which will help you to follow the meal plans and get the most benefit from them.

- Prioritise protein in each meal. Protein, and the fat that comes with it, will keep you full for longer than carbohydrates. You are aiming to consume between 0.8 and 1 g of protein per pound of your ideal weight each day. For example, if your ideal weight is 150 then you would aim for between 120 (0.8 x 150) and 150 (1 x 150) g of protein per day. You will have to research your favorite foods to find out how much protein is in different items, you can write down these figures for quick access but you will have them memorized before you know it. The shopping list which accompanies the meal plan includes the amount of protein in some of the most common sources of protein.

- Throughout this book I recommend high-quality foods such as grass-fed beef and free-range eggs. If those are within your budget, great, but if they are not, go with what you can afford. I was a student once and I remember what it was like for your entire shopping experience to be limited to the "reduced for quick sale" section.

- Only shop for that week's items – do not shop for two weeks at once as many items are perishable. The grocery lists are broken down into separate weeks.

- Try to make extra portions of the breakfasts to freeze and reheat for busier mornings when you may not have time to spend in the kitchen.

- Try to make extra portions of the dinner recipes to use for lunches the following day.

- Do not beat yourself up if you are not perfect one day; with a positive attitude you can get right back on track the next day.

- Eliminate grains (bread, pasta, crackers, and chips) from your diet as much as possible.

Snack List

Keep these foods on hand for when the urge to snack hits. Pick from these up to two times per day.

- A handful of cashews and walnuts
- A handful of pumpkin seeds with raw carrots or cucumber slices
- Sliced hard-boiled eggs on cucumber slices
- Peanut butter or almond butter on celery sticks
- Celery sticks filled with 1 can of light tuna mixed with olive oil mayonnaise
- A handful of almonds with ¼ of an avocado
- A hard-boiled egg and berries
- Gluten-free organic beef jerky with carrots
- Kale chips with almonds
- Organic hummus with carrot, celery, and cucumber slices
- A handful of pistachios and 2 kiwi fruit
- Homemade trail mix (with no dried fruit added)
- Turkey slices with zucchini sticks and cucumber slices.

Pro tip: If you are frequently hungry between meals, it may be because you are not consuming enough salt. Add a pinch of Himalayan pink salt to each glass or bottle of water you drink; this will help to keep your salt level up and provide many of the minerals you need for each day.

Week One Meal Plan

Adjust your serving size, particularly of meat, to fulfil your daily protein intake.

*The recipes for main or side dishes marked with an asterix can be found at the end of this book.

WEEK 1	BREAKFAST	SNACK	LUNCH	DINNER
DAY 1	8 oz of water with juice from ½ of a lemon Baked eggs in avocado*	1 can of light tuna mixed with olive oil on cucumber slices	Sliced chicken breast or lunch meat topped with jarred, roasted red peppers and avocado slices	Chicken and avocado salad with lime and cilantro*
DAY 2	8 oz of water with juice from ½ of a lemon Grain-free apple muffins* (Make a large batch and freeze extra portions to reheat for another day)	⅓ of a cup of cashews and ½ of a cup of fresh berries	Leftover chicken and avocado salad (from Day 1 Dinner)	Grill seasoned flank steak for about 5 minutes on each side Serve with asparagus and 1 cup of lemon poppy green beans*
DAY 3	8 oz of water with juice from ½ of a lemon Strawberry, spinach, and almond smoothie*	⅓ of a cup of pumpkin seeds and 1 cup of raw carrots	Steak "wraps"; wrap leftover steak slices (from Day 2 Dinner), red pepper, and diced tomatoes in romaine lettuce leaves	Top cod with 1 tbsp of lemon juice, sea salt, and ½ of a tsp of coconut oil; bake at 400 °F for 10–12 minutes until the fish flakes easily with a fork Serve with steamed spinach

| DAY 4 | 8 oz of water with juice from ½ of a lemon

Mini crustless vegetable quiches* (Make a large batch and freeze extra portions to reheat for another day) | Sliced hard-boiled eggs on cucumber slices | Fish "tacos"; wrap leftover fish (from Day 3 Dinner) in romaine or bibb lettuce and top with your favorite salsa | Grill grass-fed organic beef, bison, or turkey burger Serve with *no* bun; wrap in lettuce if desired and top with diced tomatoes and red onion |
|---|---|---|---|---|
| DAY 5 | 8 oz of water with juice from ½ of a lemon

Veggies and eggs Italiano* | 1 tbsp of almond butter on celery | Mix tuna, 2 slices of avocado, sliced red onion, shredded carrot, 2 tbsp of Greek yogurt, and 1 tbsp of lemon juice | Top wild salmon with 1 tsp of coconut oil, ½ of a tsp of garlic salt, and thinly sliced lemon; bake at 400°F for 15 min Serve with steamed asparagus |
| DAY 6 | 8 oz of water with juice from ½ of a lemon

2 scrambled egg whites with sautéed Swiss chard and tomatoes | ⅓ of a cup of raw almonds and ¼ of an avocado with sea salt | Leftover salmon (from Day 5 Dinner) over salad leaves Salad dressing: mix 1 tsp of coconut oil, salt, and 1 tbsp of fresh lemon juice | Grill chicken sausage Serve with grilled zucchini halves brushed with coconut or olive oil and seasoned with sea salt |

| DAY 7 | 8 oz of water with juice from ½ of a lemon

2 egg omelets, filled with sautéed mushrooms and spinach | Organic hummus with peppers, celery, and cucumbers | Leftover chicken sausage (from Day 6 Dinner) with jarred, roasted red peppers or zucchini | Pork tenderloin with peach and avocado salsa* |
|---|---|---|---|---|

Week One Grocery List

Many of the items listed below are considered pantry staples and will last for several weeks or even months, for example, spices, seeds, and dry baking ingredients. These items will not need to be replaced every week. Always buy produce that is organic and fresh, rather than packaged, where possible.

Produce:

- Organic spinach – 2 bags
- Romaine lettuce head
- Asparagus – 1 lb
- Carrots – 2 bunches
- Red or yellow peppers – 2
- Celery – 1 bunch
- Grape tomatoes – 1 container
- Red onion – 1
- Green onions – 1 bunch
- Zucchini – 2–3
- Sweet potatoes – 2
- Green Beans – ½ of a lb
- Avocados – 4
- Cucumbers – 2 or 3
- Fresh cilantro – 1 bunch
- Organic berries of choice
- Limes – 2
- Lemons – 6

- Fresh ginger
- Frozen strawberries

Poultry, Seafood, Meat, Eggs, and Dairy:

- Pastured organic eggs – 2–3 dozen
- Pre-cooked rotisserie chicken – 1 OR Boneless, skinless chicken breasts – 2 lbs
- Wild salmon fillet – 2 lbs
- Cod – 1 lb
- Pork tenderloin – 1 ½ – 2 lbs
- Sweet Italian chicken sausage – 1 ½ lbs
- Flank steak – 2 lbs
- Organic ground beef, bison, or turkey – 1 lb
- Water packed tuna – 2 cans
- Nitrite and nitrate free lunch meat – 1 package
- Bacon
- Organic, lowfat, plain Greek yogurt – 16 oz
- Coconut milk

Protein in Common Items

Eggs	6 g/egg
Steak	100 g/lb
Chicken breast	30 g
Can of sardines	23 g
Hamburger (4 oz)	30 g
Shrimp (3 oz)	20 g

Nuts, Seeds, Oils, Flours, and Spices:

- Raw pumpkin seeds
- Raw cashews
- Raw almonds
- Raw walnuts
- Almond butter – 1 jar
- Almond flour
- Chia seeds
- Poppy seeds
- Vanilla extract
- Fresh honey (preferably local)
- Cold-pressed coconut oil
- Favorite seasonings: garlic salt, paprika, etc.
- Baking soda

Miscellaneous:

- Jarred, roasted red peppers (water-packed)
- Favorite fresh salsa
- Hummus
- Raw, unfiltered apple cider vinegar
- Vanilla protein powder

Week Two Meal Plan

*The recipes for main or side dishes marked with an asterix can be found at the end of this book.

WEEK 2	BREAKFAST	SNACK	LUNCH	DINNER
DAY 1	8 oz of water with juice from ½ of a lemon 2 hard-boiled eggs, 2 slices of bacon, and fresh berries	Sliced hard-boiled eggs on cucumber slices with sea salt	Shredded rotisserie chicken salad Salad dressing; olive oil mayonnaise, 1 tsp of mustard, 1 tsp of lemon juice, diced celery, and a pinch of sea salt	Green tacos; mix 1lb of cooked ground beef or chicken seasoned with cumin, add fresh cilantro, avocado slices, tomato, & lime juice, and wrap in romaine lettuce leaves
DAY 2	8 oz of water with juice from ½ of a lemon 5-minute protein powder pancakes* (Make a large batch and freeze extra portions to reheat for another day)	⅓ of a cup of cashews and ½ of a cup of fresh berries	1 can of tuna (or chicken), raw vegetables, and spinach salad Salad dressing; 1 tbsp of fresh lemon juice	Grill chicken breast seasoned with coconut oil, sea salt, and garlic salt Serve with grilled zucchini or asparagus (Make extra portions for lunch the next day)

| DAY 3 | 8 oz of water with juice from ½ of a lemon

2 no-bake, high-energy protein bites* and fresh berries (Make a large batch and save extra portions for snacks on other days) | ⅓ of a cup of pumpkin seeds and 1 cup of raw carrots | Leftover chicken slices and vegetables (from Day 2 Dinner) on romaine lettuce leaves | Chicken meatball soup* (Make extra portions for lunch the next day) |

DAY 4	8 oz of water with juice from ½ of a lemon Veggies and eggs Italiano*	1 leftover no-bake, high-energy protein bite (from Day 3 Breakfast) or ½ of a cup of fresh berries	Leftover chicken meatball soup (from Day 3 Dinner)	Grill 1 lb of grass-fed organic beef, bison, or turkey burger Serve with *no* bun; wrap in lettuce if desired andop with real cheese, diced tomatoes, and red onion
DAY 5	8 oz of water with juice from ½ of a lemon Vegetable egg muffins*	1 cheese stick	Beef "wraps"; wrap roast beef in romaine lettuce leaves and top with horseradish, red onion, and avocado slices	Make your own fish dish*
DAY 6	8 oz of water with juice from ½ of a lemon 4 scrambled eggs with sautéed Swiss chard and tomatoes	1 can of light tuna mixed with olive oil on cucumber slices	Mix 3 oz of tuna, 2 slices of avocado, sliced red onion, shredded carrot, 2 tbsp of Greek yogurt, and 1 tbsp of lemon juice	Spaghetti squash with garlic oil*; top with ground beef, bison, turkey, or chicken, and diced tomatoes
DAY 7	8 ounces of water with juice from ½ of a lemon Strawberry, spinach, and almond smoothie*	Hummus with carrots, celery, and cucumbers	Sliced chicken breast or lunch meat topped with jarred, roasted red peppers and avocado slices	"Easiest Roast Chicken Dinner" * (Save leftover chicken for lunch the next day)

Adjust your serving size, particularly of meat, to fulfil your daily protein intake.

Week Two Grocery List

Remember, many of the items were on Week One's Grocery List. Take stock of your leftover ingredients before your shopping trip.

Produce:

- Organic spinach – 2 bags
- Romaine lettuce head
- Swiss chard – 1 bunch
- Asparagus – 1 lb
- Carrots – 2–3 bunches
- Red peppers – 2
- Celery – 1 bunch
- Grape tomatoes – 1 container
- Plum tomatoes – 1 container
- Red onion – 1
- Onion – 1
- Green onions – 1 bunch
- Zucchini – 2–3
- Sweet potatoes – 2
- Spaghetti squash – 1
- Avocados – 4
- Cucumbers – 2–3
- Fresh cilantro – 1 bunch
- Fresh basil
- Organic berries of choice
- Kiwis – 2
- Apples – 2
- Limes – 2
- Lemons – 2
- Frozen strawberries

Poultry, Seafood, Meat, Eggs, and Dairy:

- Pastured organic eggs – 2–3 dozen
- Pre-cooked rotisserie chicken – 1 OR Boneless, skinless chicken breasts – 2 lbs
- Your choice of wild fish – 2 lbs (salmon, ahi, mahi-mahi, swordfish, or snapper)
- Organic ground beef, bison, or turkey – 2 lbs
- Ground chicken – 2 lbs
- Water packed tuna – 2 cans
- Nitrite and nitrate free roast beef lunch meat – 1 package
- Bacon
- Organic, full-fat, plain greek yogurt – 16 oz
- Coconut milk

Nuts, Seeds, Oils, Flours, and Spices:

- Raw pumpkin seeds
- Raw cashews
- Raw almonds
- Raw walnuts
- Almond butter – 1 jar
- Almond flour
- Chia seeds
- Hemp seeds
- Raw cacao powder

- Vanilla extract
- Fresh honey (preferably local)
- Cold-pressed coconut oil
- Favorite seasonings: garlic salt, paprika, cinnamon, etc.
- Baking soda

Miscellaneous:

- Jarred, roasted red peppers (water-packed)
- Favorite fresh salsa
- Fresh horseradish sauce
- Hummus
- Gluten-free, organic chicken broth – 32 oz
- Gluten-free chicken bullion cubes
- Raw, unfiltered apple cider vinegar
- Vanilla protein powder

7

TIME YOUR EATING AND EXERCISE TO HEAL YOUR FATTY LIVER

The diet changes recommended in the Fatty Liver Diet Protocol will be most effective when they are supported by thoughtful meal timings and regular exercise. I recommend intermittent fasting and high intensity interval training as the best strategies to maximize the effectiveness of your diet. Changes in diet, intermittent fasting, and high-intensity interval training combined create a lifestyle which will boost your health and wellbeing, and prevent and combat fatty liver disease.

INTERMITTENT FASTING

Intermittent Fasting (known as IF) is not a diet in itself; it is an eating pattern which incorporates voluntary fasting. It involves alternating cycles of fasting and eating; it does not restrict the types of foods that you can eat, instead it provides a guideline of when you should eat them.

If you are intermittent fasting, you will only eat during a specific time of the day. Fasting for a certain number of hours each day can help your body burn fat. It works by extending the length of time your body has to burn through the calories consumed during your last meal and triggering your body to begin burning fat.

Incorporating intermittent fasting into your eating routine allows your body to detoxify more efficiently. It also helps you to better understand feelings of hunger. Fasting causes a metabolic shift that helps the body to more effectively regenerate, eliminate waste, and repair cells.

During your fasting periods, you are only allowed to consume water and beverages with no calories, such as tea or black coffee. During your eating periods, you should consume foods and meals that are recommended in this book. Fasting in this way will allow you to better understand feelings of hunger.

BENEFITS OF INTERMITTENT FASTING

There are many health benefits associated with intermittent fasting.

Weight Loss

Intermittent fasting promotes weight loss; particularly weight loss around the belly. This is especially important when you have a fatty liver because fat tends to accumulate in the belly region. Reducing and removing this fat is crucial when you are trying to repair liver damage.

Improved Blood Sugar Levels and Insulin Resistance

Intermittent fasting has been shown to counter insulin resistance; therefore, it can also help to reduce blood sugar levels and avoid or reverse the effects of type 2 diabetes. Insulin resistance, high blood sugar levels, and type 2 diabetes are all known risk factors which contribute to the development of fatty liver disease; combating these metabolic conditions is key to repairing liver damage.

Oxidative Stress

Oxidative stress is when free radicals in the body damage healthy cells and waste products build up. Intermittent fasting can help to prevent oxidative stress by reducing inflammation in the cells, suppressing cell growth to prevent the formation of certain cancers, and protecting the cells from DNA damage.

Gut Healing

Intermittent fasting can help to increase the amount of good bacteria in the gut and decrease the amount of bad bacteria. Fasting gives your digestive system a period of rest. During this time, your gut is able to heal and this helps to prevent "leaky gut" which can lead to other conditions such as Crohn's disease and Irritable Bowel Syndrome.

How to Follow an Intermittent Fasting Schedule

There are several different intermittent fasting methods, but they are all based on choosing regular time periods to eat and fast. I will describe four of the different intermittent fasting schedules you can follow. Each method has its own benefits. Pick the method that you feel would be the easiest for you to follow and will best suit your own schedule and routine. It is also important to speak with your doctor to make sure that intermittent fasting is safe for you to do.

12–12 Fast

A twelve-hour fast simply means that you should eat for twelve hours during the day and then fast for the remaining twelve. This is the best way to begin an intermittent fasting schedule. You can slowly add an hour a day to your fasting window as you grow accustomed to eating this way. This method is fairly easy to stick to, and thus great for beginners, but may not be optimal for weight loss.

16–8 Fast

As you become comfortable with fasting, you can increase your fasting window to sixteen hours. A common approach to this fast is to eat your first meal of the day at noon and finish your last meal at 8pm. After 8pm you would consume nothing but calorie-free liquids until the next day at noon. You can pick the meal times that work best for you with this method as long as you are fasting for sixteen hours and keeping your eating window within the remaining eight hours.

5–2 Fast

This approach to intermittent fasting is daily rather than hourly; it involves eating regularly for five days of the week and then drastically restricting calorie intake for the other two days. This is a popular method of intermittent fasting because you can eat normally for five days of the week without having to change your routine. On the other two days you restrict your calorie intake to 25% of your regular daily intake. The term "fasting" is a little misleading; you are still eating on your fasting days, just a limited amount. With this method, it is important that your fasting days are not consecutive because you need to give your body the calories and nutrients it needs to function optimally.

Alternate Day Fasting

This approach involves fasting every other day. It is similar to the 5–2 method; on fasting days you limit your calorie consumption to about 25% of your usual intake and on your regular, non-fasting days you eat normally. Some stricter approaches to this method say that you should consume no calories on your fasting days, but this is very severe and is not usually recommended.

Overall, it is important to remain consistent with whichever method you choose. You can try the different fasting times and approaches to decide which one feels most natural to you and which one you will be able to commit to in the long term. While every method can be effective, it really comes down to which one works best for you. No matter which approach you choose, the most important thing is to ensure that you are consuming high quality foods packed full of nutrients when you are actually eating. Following the food suggestions in this book will keep you on track during intermittent fasting and allow you to optimize your liver health.

HIGH-INTENSITY INTERVAL TRAINING (HIIT)

Exercise is crucial for optimal liver health. It is essential for weight loss, which you should know by now has a very positive impact on liver health; basically, the more weight you lose, the healthier your liver will become. Moving in any way will be beneficial to your liver health, but certain forms of physical activity are more effective than others at reducing fat cells in the liver.

One of the most effective forms of exercise to target a fatty liver is High-Intensity Interval Training (most commonly known as HIIT). HIIT describes any workout that alternates between intense bursts of physical activity and periods of less intense activity. It usually involves several minutes of intense movements followed by lower-intensity recovery periods.

HIIT workouts can definitely pack a punch; they are far more effective in shorter amounts of time than a typical, moderate form of exercise. You can get an extremely beneficial workout in as little as ten minutes. A typical HIIT workout can last between 10–30 minutes and includes a variety of different forms of exercise.

The biggest key to your HIIT workouts being effective, however, is how *intense* your intense intervals actually are. You cannot just give 50% of your energy during these periods; this form of workout is designed for you to work as hard as you can.The premise of this form of exercise is that you are challenging yourself to expend the maximum amount of energy possible, and then mixing these bursts of intensity with periods of recovery.

Benefits of HITT

In addition to reducing liver fat, HIIT has many other extremely useful and attractive benefits.

1. It is efficient

HIIT workouts are one of the most effective workouts for anyone who has very limited time to exercise. The average workout takes between 20–30 minutes, but they can be extremely effective in as little as 10 minutes. You can get more benefits from a HIIT workout in 10–15 minutes than you can from an entire hour of jogging. It is one of the most effective ways to get your heart rate up and tap into the fat burning zone.

2. You can workout anywhere

The hallmark of HIIT is simply short bursts of intense exercise that get your heart rate up, so any type of exercise can qualify. Whether it is sprinting, swimming, jump roping, playing tennis, squat jumps, or burpees, as long as it gets your heart rate up fast, it qualifies. You do not need any equipment, and you can modify workouts to fit any time or space constraints you have. This means that even when you are traveling, stuck in your office at work, or home while the kids are napping, you can still workout effectively. With HITT there are no barriers to getting into shape and losing weight.

3. Your body will become a fat-burning machine

HIIT workouts are ideal for burning fat and building lean muscle (which continues the cycle of burning even more fat). The anaerobic part of HIIT workouts forces your body to use energy from stored fats, instead of carbohydrates, which makes fat burning more efficient. You will continue to burn fat long after you are done exercising for the day because the intense exertion keeps your body in fat-burning mode.

4. Your metabolism will increase

Not only will your fat burning be kicked into high gear, your metabolism will also increase due to the stimulation of the production of Human Growth Hormone (HGH). HGH spikes after a HIIT workout, which increases your metabolism and your overall metabolic rate. This, in turn, improves insulin resistance and leads to weight loss. A healthy metabolic system will also help you get rid of toxins from your liver more efficiently and eliminate them from your body. These metabolic effects will last for hours after you have finished your HITT workout.

Simple HIIT Workouts You Can Do Anywhere

Here are some examples of simple workouts that can be done in your living room, your backyard, a local park, or even a hotel room if you are traveling. They require little to no equipment and not much space at all.

Jump Rope Interval Workout

Directions: Complete the following circuit four times, resting for one min in between each round.

1. Jump rope – 1 min
2. Push-ups from your knees – 20–30 repetitions
3. Mountain climbers – 45 reps (count each time your knee comes towards your elbow as one rep)
4. Plank – 1 min
5. High knees – 30 secs

Lower-Body Interval Workout

Directions: Complete the following circuit four times, resting for one min after the calf raises in each round. This is best suited to a backyard or a park.

1. Sprint – 30 seconds
2. Squat jumps – 45 secs
3. Lunges – 20 each leg
4. Calf Raises – 50 repetitions
5. Skater Jumps – 10 each leg

Burpee Interval Workout

Directions: Complete the following circuit four times, resting for one min after the burpees in each round.

1. Push-ups – as many repetitions as possible in 30 secs
2. Jumping Jacks – 60 repetitions
3. Burpees – 20 repetitions

20-Minute AMRAP

Directions: Complete As Many Rounds as Possible (AMRAP) within 20 minutes.

1. Reverse lunges – 10 each leg
2. Bear crawl – travel 15 ft
3. Walking lunges – 1o each leg
4. Squat jumps – 15 repetitions

Will HIIT Heal a Fatty Liver?

As you can see, these workouts can be done by anyone, anywhere. You don't have to spend a lot of money on a gym membership; you can find thousands of videos online to follow, or you can stick to the simple exercises that I have included here. Start slowly, build up your endurance, and I truly believe that you will amaze yourself with what you can accomplish. As your workouts get easier for you, challenge yourself to work harder or to do more difficult exercises. Your confidence will soar as you get stronger, feel better, have more energy, and begin to lose weight.

While exercise alone will not deliver all of the healing results your liver needs, it is definitely one of the key pieces of the puzzle. When you pair physical activity with optimal nutrition, plenty of sleep, and stress reduction, you will transform your body, your health, and your energy. You have the power to unlock the healthy version of yourself that has been hiding all of this time. By transforming your workout routine, your nutrition, and even your stress levels, you will be transforming your life for good as well.

Now that you have an understanding of the power of simple, short bursts of exercise that you can squeeze in anytime and anywhere, you can appreciate that you will have plenty of time to focus on a balanced and colorful diet; one that is brimming with vegetables, protein, healthy fats, and plenty of water. My hope is that you now see that this formula is really simple and far less intimidating than it may have initially seemed to you. There is absolutely no reason to get overwhelmed, I am giving you everything that you need. You have a blueprint to follow: meal plans, grocery lists, and workouts.

8

RECIPES FOR THE FATTY LIVER DIET PROTOCOL

The following recipes are all meant to be simple enough for even the most novice of cooks to follow without feeling overwhelmed. Most of these recipes require very few ingredients and very little time, and will allow you to put a meal on the table that the entire family will enjoy. You can feel good about the fact that you are making great strides towards healing your own fatty liver with these nutrient dense meals while also encouraging your entire family to become healthier at the same time.

SMOOTHIES

Strawberry, spinach, and almond smoothie

Ingredients:

1 cup of whole milk (or a higher protein milk, for example, Fairlife)

¼–½ of a cup of frozen, chopped spinach

3–4 large strawberries (frozen or fresh)

½ of an avocado

2–3 heaping tbsp of raw almond butter

Directions:

Mix all ingredients together in a blender for 20–30 seconds.

Berry and ginger smoothie

Ingredients:

1 ½ cups of frozen berries

1 cup of ice

½ of a cup of full-fat, plain Greek yogurt

2 tsp of fresh ginger (peeled and chopped)

Juice from ½ of a lemon

Leaves from 1 sprig of mint

Directions:

Mix all ingredients together in a blender for 20–30 seconds.

Liver detox smoothie

Ingredients:

½ of an avocado

½ of a green apple (cored and chopped)

1 medium-sized carrot (peeled and chopped)

1 handful of baby spinach

1 (¼ in) nub of turmeric root (peeled)

1 tbsp of fresh parsley (chopped)

3 walnut halves

2 tbsp of hemp protein powder

Juice from ½ of a lemon

1 pinch of cinnamon (optional)

½ a teaspoon of honey (optional)

¾ of a cup of whole milk

Directions:

Mix ingredients together in a blender and blend until completely smooth. Taste smoothie for flavor and add 1 pinch of cinnamon or ½ of a teaspoon of honey to taste.

Green machine smoothie

Ingredients:

1 cup of baby spinach

1 cup of kale or chard

½ of a cup of broccoli sprouts

1 carrot (chopped)

2 tbsp of almonds or walnuts

½ of an avocado

Filtered water (as needed)

Directions:

Mix all ingredients together in a blender and puree until smooth. Add filtered water as needed to create desired consistency.

Ginger, berry and greens smoothie

Ingredients:

3 tbsp of hemp protein powder

2 in piece of fresh, raw ginger (peeled)

2 cups of leafy greens (kale, collards, romaine, spinach, chard, etc.)

1 cup of celery

1 cup of mixed frozen berries (strawberries, blueberries, cranberries, etc.)

½ of a cup of filtered water

Directions:

Mix all ingredients together in a blender for 1 min or until desired consistency is reached.

Protein power smoothie

Ingredients:

½ of a cup of frozen berries (strawberries, blueberries, cranberries, etc.)

½ of a cup of fresh greens (kale, collards, romaine, spinach, chards)

1 cup of whole milk

1 scoop of vanilla protein powder

1 scoop of powdered greens

1–2 tbsp of chia seeds (optional source of additional Omega 3s)

Directions:

Mix all ingredients together in a blender until desired consistency is reached.

Healing green juice

Ingredients:

4 large kale leaves (stems removed)

⅓ of a medium-sized cucumber

½ of a lemon

⅓ of a green apple

3 tsp of raw honey

¼ in piece fresh, raw ginger (peeled)

3 cups of filtered water

1 cup of ice

Directions:

For Blender: Mix all ingredients together in a blender until smooth.

For Juicer: Add all ingredients to a juicer in the order listed above, minus the water and ice.

Serve over ice.

Energy boosting juice

Ingredients:

½ of a red or golden beet (cut to fit through juicer)

½ of a medium-sized cucumber (cut to fit through juicer)

½ of a lemon (peeled)

2 celery stalks

1 handful of cilantro

1 handful of chard

1 in piece of ginger (peeled)

3 cups of filtered water

1 cup of ice

Directions:

For blender: Mix all ingredients together in a blender until smooth.

For juicer: Add all ingredients to a juicer in the order listed above, minus the water and ice.

Serve over ice.

BREAKFAST

Baked eggs in avocado

Ingredients:

2 ripe avocados

4 fresh, pastured organic eggs

⅛ of a tsp of salt

⅛ of a tsp pf pepper

1 tbsp of fresh basil (slivered)

Directions:

1. Preheat the oven to 425 °F.

2. Slice the avocados in half, and remove the pit. Scoop out two tablespoons of flesh from the center of the avocado, just enough so that the egg will fit snugly in the center.

3. Place the avocado halves in a small baking dish. Crack an egg into each avocado half; add yolk first, then let the egg whites fill up the rest of the avocado.

4. Place in the oven and bake for 15 to 20 mins: cooking time will depend on the size of your eggs and avocados, make sure the egg whites have enough time to set.

5. Remove from the oven and top with slivered basil.

Easy vegetable and egg Italiano

INGREDIENTS:

¼ of a cup of distilled white vinegar

2 tsp of extra-virgin olive oil

1 shallot or small onion (minced)

1 garlic clove (minced)

1 lb of zucchini (diced)

3–4 plum tomatoes (diced)

3 tbsp of thinly sliced fresh basil

1 tbsp of balsamic vinegar

½ of a tsp of salt

½ of a tsp of freshly ground pepper (optional)

8 fresh, pastured eggs

2 tbsp of freshly grated Parmesan cheese

Directions:

1. Fill a large, straight-sided skillet or Dutch oven with 2 in of water; bring to a boil and add white vinegar.

2. Heat the oil in a large non-stick skillet over a medium-high heat. Add the shallot and garlic and cook, stirring for about 1 min until fragrant. Stir in the zucchini and tomatoes and cook for about ten mins until the zucchini is tender, stirring occasionally. Remove from the heat and stir in the basil, balsamic vinegar, salt and pepper.

3. Reduce the boiling water (from Step 1.) to a gentle simmer; the water should be steaming and small bubbles should come up from the bottom of the pan. Crack the eggs into a small bowl and slip them into the simmering water one at a time, taking care not to break the yolks. Cook for 4 mins for soft-set, 5 mins for medium-set, and 8 mins for hard-set eggs. Once cooked, use a slotted spoon to transfer the eggs to a clean kitchen towel to drain.

4. To serve, place some of the vegetable mixture, an egg,

a sprinkling of cheese, and the remaining basil onto a plate.

Vegetable egg muffins

Ingredients:

1 cup of frozen or fresh spinach (chopped)

8 fresh, pastured eggs

¼ of a cup of whole milk

½ of a cup of diced tomato

¼ of a tsp of salt

¼ of a tsp of pepper

¼ of a tsp paprika

Fresh herbs (basil, oregano, marjoram, etc.; slivered)

Directions:

1. Preheat the oven to 375 degrees °F. Arrange spinach on the bottoms of a paper-lined muffin pan (approximately 1 tbsp per cup).
2. Add a thin layer of diced tomato to each cup. Season with salt and pepper. Beat the eggs in a small bowl with the milk and additional salt and pepper. Spoon the egg mix into each cup; fill almost to the top and sprinkle with paprika and fresh herbs.
3. Bake for 15–20 mins (check after 15 mins and continue to cook if required). Save any extras for other

mornings when you do not have time to prepare breakfast.

Mini crustless vegetable quiches

Ingredients:

1 cup of frozen or fresh spinach (chopped)

8 pastured, organic eggs

¼ of a cup of plain coconut milk

½ of a cup of diced tomato

¼ of a tsp of salt

¼ of a tsp of pepper

¼ of a tsp of paprika

4 slices of cooked and crumbled bacon

Directions:

1. Preheat the oven to 375 °F. Arrange spinach on the bottoms of a paper-lined muffin pan (approximately 1 tbsp per cup). Add a thin layer of diced tomato to each cup and season with salt and pepper.

2. Beat the eggs in a small bowl with milk and additional salt and pepper. Spoon the egg mix into each cup; fill almost to the top and sprinkle with paprika and bacon. Bake for 15–20 mins (check after 15 mins and continue to cook if necessary). Save any extras for other

mornings when you do not have time to prepare breakfast; these freeze well.

No-bake, high-energy protein bites

Ingredients:

- 1 cup of almond flour
- 3 tbsp of ground chia seeds
- 3 tbsp of hemp seeds
- 2 tbsp of raw cacao powder
- 1 tsp of cinnamon
- ¼ of a tsp of salt
- ⅔ of a cup of almond butter
- 2 tsp of raw honey (if needed)
- 2 tsp of vanilla extract
- 2 tsp of chopped pumpkin seeds

Directions:

1. In a large bowl, combine the oats, ground chia, hemp seeds, cacao powder, cinnamon, and salt. Add in the almond butter, maple syrup, vanilla, and pumpkin seeds
2. Scoop 1 tbsp of the mixture and roll it between your hands to make a ball. Place on a cookie sheet. Repeat until all of the mixture is used; this recipe should make about 20–28 bites.

3. Place the cookie sheet in the refrigerator for about 30 mins to set. Once chilled, store in an airtight container in the refrigerator for up to 1 week. Pair with hard-boiled eggs for a great grab-and-go meal.

Grain-free apple muffins

Ingredients:

2 cups of almond flour (almond meal)

3 fresh, pastured eggs

2 tbsp of melted, grass-fed butter

2 tbsp of honey

2 tsp of ground cinnamon

1–2 apples (cored)

1 tsp of baking soda

⅛ of a tsp of salt

Directions:

1. Preheat the oven to 325 °F.
2. Blend cored apple(s) until finely chopped, but not pureed. Mix all ingredients together in a bowl.
3. Line a muffin pan with paper and then fill each of the cups until ¾ full.
4. Bake for 20 mins. This recipe makes around 10 muffins.

5-minute protein powder pancakes

Ingredients:

4 fresh, pastured eggs

1 cup of unsweetened whole milk or coconut water

½ of an avocado

1 tbsp of vanilla extract

2 ¼ cups of blanched almond flour

2 tsp of baking soda

¼ of a tsp of salt

Fresh berries

1 tbsp of coconut oil for cooking

Directions:

1. In your food processor or blender, mix together the eggs, milk (or coconut water), and avocado until smooth. Add the almond flour, baking soda, and salt to create a batter.
2. Heat some of the coconut oil in a large skillet, and add the batter to make 3–4 in diameter pancakes. Cook for approximately 3 mins until they are golden on the bottom and the pancake wants to flip easily (when bubbles start to appear and pop). You can add the berries to the pancakes before flipping, if desired.
3. Flip the pancakes and cook for a further 2 mins. Add more oil as necessary. Enjoy topped with fresh berries.

LUNCH

Instead of specific recipes, here are some simple lunch suggestions that are easy to prepare and can be made in advance and served over several days.

- **Leftovers from breakfast** – for example, mini egg quiches or no-bake, high-energy protein bars.
- **Nori (seaweed) wraps** – where seaweed is used as a substitute for a tortilla wrap or bread; serve with your favorite meat and vegetables.
- **Lettuce sandwiches or wraps** – where lettuce is used as a substitute for a tortilla wrap or bread; serve with your favorite meat and vegetables.
- **Tuna-stuffed deviled eggs.**
- **Egg salad** with a side of berries.
- **Superfood salad** – start with a leafy green, like spinach or kale, and add a chopped vegetable of every color (red/yellow/orange bell peppers, tomatoes, onion, cucumber, celery, carrots, etc.). Add high-Omega 3 nuts or seeds for crunch (walnuts, pumpkin seeds, etc.) and a superfruit like pomegranate seeds or berries. Mix a little extra virgin olive oil and apple cider vinegar for the dressing. Top with grilled chicken, hard boiled eggs, smoked turkey breast, or another lean meat. Prep all of your vegetables and meat

on the day you buy them so all you have to do is
assemble the salad at mealtime.

- **Healthy chicken salad** – instead of mayonnaise,
  use a combination of avocado and plain, organic Greek
  yogurt to make a chicken salad dressing (I like to add
  celery, green and red onions, cilantro, and lime juice).
  Serve on a bed of leafy greens or lettuce cups, or use a
  collard green leaf as a wrap.

- **Quinoa salad** – prepare quinoa (you can do this
  ahead of time and store in the fridge) and season with
  your favorite spices and fresh herbs. Mix together
  chopped vegetables (asparagus, cherry tomatoes, bell
  peppers, artichokes, etc.), lean meat, and avocado. (For
  a simple and healthy dressing, see the example above
  or the recipes included in the Dinner section.)

- **Soup** – make a large batch of your favorite soup to eat
  throughout the week (soup recipes are included in the
  following section.)

- **Burrito bowl** – prepare cauliflower rice, add roasted
  red peppers, lean meat or seafood (like shrimp), and
  mix with salsa or fire roasted tomatoes. Top with
  avocado and a splash of lime juice.

- **Turkey burger** – mix together ground turkey breast
  with hatch chiles and seasoning; form into a patty and
  grill. Serve in a large piece of bibb lettuce or on a bed
  of spinach. Top with tomato, onion, and sliced

avocado. You can also make these ahead of time, and then freeze and reheat.

- **Veggie pizza** – layer wilted spinach, fresh basil, minced garlic, caramelized onions, thinly-sliced tomatoes or sun-dried tomatoes, fire roasted red peppers, and cubed chicken onto a premade cauliflower pizza crust. Top with shredded mozzarella cheese. Bake in the oven at 400 °F for 10 mins.

- **Beef and broccoli** – take leftover or pre-prepared beef (such as grass-fed flank steak), toss with baked spaghetti squash (or wilted bean sprouts), steamed broccoli, sesame seeds, coconut oil, white wine vinegar, fish sauce, chopped green onions, shredded carrots, and chopped peanuts.

- **Leftovers from dinner the night before**.

HEALING SOUPS

Bone Broth

Bone broth has a long history of being used in traditional Chinese culture; it has many health benefits and healing properties, including aiding digestion, because it is rich in collagen, minerals, amino acids, and compounds found in bones and connective tissues. It is one of the most nutritious and cost-effective foods that you can make for yourself at home. It is full of protein and is both healing and restorative. It can be used as a base in soups, stews, or any meal that includes broth or liquid. It is often sipped straight from a mug all by itself.

Bone broth is made by simmering the bones of animals for hours and hours (often over 20 hours), along with vegetables for flavor and something acidic, like vinegar, to draw the minerals and nutrients out from the bone and marrow. The end result is a savory and nutrient-dense liquid.

It is hard to think of anyone who could not benefit from bone broth; but, if you are struggling with a fatty liver, leaky gut symptoms, Irritable Bowel Diseases (IBD), like Crohn's or Ulcerative Colitis, or a sluggish digestion, then you will definitely feel the advantages of consuming more bone broth. Bone broth has also been found to help with food allergies, aching joints, and low energy.

Benefits of Bone Broth

There are a huge number of health benefits associated with consuming more bone broth.

1. **Promotes healing**: has been used successfully in treating gastro-intestinal disorders, including hyper-acidity, colitis, Crohn's disease, and infant diarrhea.
2. **Digestive aid**: aids in the digestibility of grains, beans, legumes, vegetables, and meats, and is hydrophilic in nature.
3. **Macro minerals**: contains highly absorbable forms

of calcium, magnesium, potassium, phosphorus, sulfur, and fluoride, as well as trace minerals.

4. **Gelatin and Collagen**: rich in both and promotes bone and joint healing in addition to supporting digestion; particularly broths made from the feet of chickens.

5. **Protein**: adds easily digestible protein to your diet.

6. **Amino acids**: aids in the formation of glycine, proline, hydroxyproline, and lysine, which are important for detoxification and amino acid production in the body.

7. **Joint support**: produces glucosamine, chondroitin sulfate, and hyaluronic acid, and provides additional muscle and joint support.

8. **Immune system**: promotes the assimilation of vitamins and minerals and thus supports the immune system.

9. **Delicious and nutritious**: can be used as a soup, cooking liquid, sauce, or as tea.

Bone Broth Recipe

Ingredients:

1 chicken carcass (previously roasted) OR 2 to 3 lbs of bony chicken parts (feet, necks, backs, breastbones, and

wings); *organic, free-range chickens yields most gelatinous stocks*

Gizzards from one chicken (optional)

2–4 chicken feet (optional)

4 qts of cold, filtered water

2 tbsp of apple cider vinegar

1 large onion (coarsely chopped; leave the peel on for a golden color in stock)

2 carrots (peeled and coarsely chopped)

2 parsnips (peeled and coarsely chopped)

2 turnips (peeled and coarsely chopped)

3 celery stalks (coarsely chopped)

3 garlic cloves(whole)

1 in piece of ginger

1 bunch of parsley

Filtered water

Directions:

1. Put the chicken bones in a large stock pot and cover completely with the cold, filtered water. Add apple cider vinegar, all of the vegetables, the garlic, and the ginger. Let it sit for 1 hr without turning the stove on.

2. Bring the stock to a boil (barely), and remove the scum that is rising to the top. Reduce the heat and let it simmer for 18 to 24 hrs (the longer you leave it the better; this

allows the gelatin to be released from the bones and gives much more flavor to the broth). At the end of your cooking time (during the last 15 mins), add your parsley and any additional fresh vegetables for a last hit of flavor.

3. Strain the stock through a fine mesh sieve into a bowl or glass container. Once strained, place the container into the refrigerator and allow the top layer of fat to congeal; remove this layer of fat and pour the remaining stock into containers (quilted, glass mason jars work wonderfully for this).

You can use your bone broth when you are making rice, pastas, sauces, soups, stews, or drink it straight from a mug. You can season depending on the recipe you are using. Consume as much broth as possible during your day, especially during the healing phase of your fatty liver disease.

OTHER SOUP RECIPES

Kale, cabbage, and bean soup

Ingredients:

2 tbsp of olive oil or coconut oil

1 sweet onion (coarsely chopped)

1 yellow Hannah sweet potato (peeled and diced into 1 in cubes)

3 carrots or parsnips or a combination of both (peeled and sliced diagonally)

4–6 garlic cloves (minced)

5 cups of bone broth (seasoned with salt and pepper)

2–3 tsp of Italian seasoning

1 tsp of garlic salt

14 ½ oz can of diced tomatoes, with juice

1 can of cannellini or northern beans (drained and rinsed well)

3 cups of kale leaves (thinly sliced and tough stems removed)

3 cups of green cabbage (thinly sliced)

½ of a cup of fresh basil leaves (thinly sliced; for garnish)

½ of a tsp of salt

½ of a tsp of pepper

Directions:

1. Heat the oil in a large stockpot. Add onion, sweet potato cubes, and carrot and/or parsnip pieces, and sauté for 5 mins. Add garlic and cook for a further 1–2 mins, stirring occasionally.

2. Add broth, Italian seasoning, and garlic salt, and bring to a boil. Reduce the heat to a simmer and cover the pot; cook for 35 mins, or until the vegetables begin to soften.

3. Stir in tomatoes, beans, kale, and cabbage, and allow to

return to a boil. Reduce heat and cook for another 10–15 mins. Season with salt and pepper.

4. Serve into bowls and top each bowl with 1–2 tbsp of the fresh basil.

Easy meatball soup

Ingredients:

1 tbsp of olive oil

½ of an onion (finely chopped)

2 garlic cloves

10 carrots (sliced into thin circles)

2 celery stalks

4 cups of bone broth

1 beef or chicken bullion cube, or vegetable bullion (gluten free)

½ of a lb of ground beef or chicken meat

Directions:

1. Heat the oil in a large stock pot. Add the garlic, onions, carrots, and celery, and cook for about 5 mins. Add the bone broth and bring to a boil. Add bullion if desired.

2. While waiting for the broth to come to a boil, scoop up small amounts of ground meat and make into little balls. When the broth is boiling carefully add in the meatballs.

3. Reduce to a simmer and add bullion if desired. Cook for about 7 mins or until the meatballs are done; take one out and cut it in half just to be sure.

Coconut and ginger vegetable soup

Ingredients:

4 cups of water (spring, filtered or distilled)

3 zucchini (chopped)

2 tomatoes (chopped)

3 celery stalks (diced)

1 carrot (finely diced)

1 large bunch of fresh parsley (stems and leaves roughly chopped)

1 cup of chopped kale

1 cup of organic canned coconut milk

4–5 garlic cloves (minced)

1 in piece of fresh ginger (peeled and grated)

2 tsp of dried oregano

1 tsp of salt

1 tsp of black pepper

Directions:

1. Add all of the ingredients, except for the kale and coconut milk, to a medium pot. Bring to a boil, reduce

the heat, cover the pot, and simmer for 30 mins or until the carrots are tender.

2. Add the kale and coconut milk to the pot and simmer until the kale is wilted, for about 3 mins. Season with salt and pepper.

Liver detox cabbage soup

Ingredients:

1 tbsp of coconut oil or ghee
½ of a small cabbage (sliced thinly)
3 stalks of celery (chopped)
½ of a tsp of salt
2 cloves of garlic (minced)
½ – 1 tsp of grated fresh ginger
2 ½ cups of bone broth
1 cup of leftover chicken, or any lean meat that you prefer (chopped or shredded)
Fresh cilantro for garnish

Directions:

1. Melt coconut oil or ghee in a soup pot over a medium–high heat. Add cabbage, celery, and salt. Saute for 3–4 mins or until the vegetables start to soften, and stir often. Add garlic and ginger and cook for another min.

2. Add the bone broth and chicken to the pot and simmer until the vegetables are cooked to your liking.

3. Garnish with fresh cilantro and serve immediately. Store leftovers in an airtight glass container for up to 2 days.

DINNER

Recipes in this section are intended to serve a family of four but can be adjusted to feed more or less people or to provide larger or smaller portions.

Chicken and avocado salad with lime and cilantro

Ingredients:

2 medium avocados (diced)

1 tbsp of fresh lime juice

½ of a tsp of salt

1 tbsp of fresh lemon juice

2 tbsp of olive oil mayonnaise

2 cups of cooked chicken breasts OR 1 cooked rotisserie chicken (diced or shredded into large pieces)

3 tbsp of green onions (thinly sliced)

⅓ of a cup of fresh cilantro (finely chopped)

½ of a cup of cherry tomatoes (slice in half)

½ of a tsp of salt

Directions:

1. Toss the diced avocado pieces with the lime juice and salt. In a separate bowl, mix lemon juice and mayonnaise for the dressing.
2. Place diced or shredded chicken in a large bowl, add the avocado mixture and dressing (from Step 1.) and the green onion slices, and toss together until the chicken is coated.
3. Add the cilantro and cherry tomatoes and toss again until just barely coated. Taste for seasoning and add more salt if needed. Serve fresh or chill in the fridge for later.

Pork tenderloin with peach and avocado salsa

Ingredients:

½ lb pork tenderloin

⅓ of a cup of balsamic vinegar

1 tsp of raw honey

3 tbsp of white wine

½ of a teaspoon of salt

1 avocado (diced)

2 peaches (sliced) OR 1 mango (diced)

1 red onion (finely chopped)

2 tbsp of fresh dill (chopped)

½ of a tsp of salt

½ of a tsp of pepper

Directions:

1. Preheat the oven to 375 °F. Place the pork in a resealable ziplock bag. In a bowl, combine the balsamic vinegar, honey, white wine, and half of the salt; whisk to combine, then pour the mixture over the pork to marinate for about 30 mins (or overnight).

2. While the pork is marinating, combine the avocado, peaches, red onion, dill, and salt in a bowl to create a salsa and set aside.

3. Remove the pork from the marinade and place the pork in a small roasting pan. Pour the remaining marinade from the bag over the pork, then cover the pan with foil. Roast for 15 mins, covered; then remove the foil and roast uncovered for another 5–10 mins, or until the internal temperature is about 140 °F.

4. Slice the pork into thin medallions and drizzle with the juices from the pan. Serve with salsa.

The easiest roast chicken dinner

Ingredients:

5 lb chicken

4 tbsp of extra virgin olive oil or softened butter

2 yellow onions (roughly chopped)

3 lbs of yellow potatoes (diced into 1 in pieces)

4 large carrots (peeled and chopped into 1 in pieces)

4 garlic cloves (mashed)

2 tsp of garlic salt

2 tsp of smoked paprika

5 tsp of salt

Directions:

1. Preheat the oven to 400 degrees °F. Place the chicken in a large roasting pan or baking dish. In a small bowl, mix together the olive oil or butter, half of the garlic salt, and the mashed garlic. Rub the mixture generously over the entire chicken, including under the skin on the breast. Season the entire chicken generously with half of the salt and half of the smoked paprika. Tie the legs of chicken together.

2. Place the pan on the middle shelf of the oven and roast for 30 mins.

3. Pull the roasting pan out and scatter the onions, potatoes, and carrots around the chicken, and season with the remaining salt, garlic salt, and smoked paprika. Roast for another 30 mins at 375 °F.

4. Cover the chicken *loosely* with foil to prevent over-browning and cook for another 25–30 mins, or until the chicken is cooked through.

5. Let the chicken sit for 15 mins before carving. Serve with the vegetables.

Grilled chicken breast with roasted peppers

Ingredients:

2 lbs of boneless, skinless chicken breasts

2 red, yellow, or orange bell peppers (sliced in quarters and seeds removed)

3 tbsp of coconut oil

1 tsp of smoked paprika

¾ of a tsp of salt

¾ of a tsp of pepper

Directions:

1. Preheat the grill to a medium–high heat. Pour coconut oil evenly over the chicken breasts and sliced pepper season with smoked paprika, salt, and pepper.
2. Place the chicken and peppers on the grill and cook for about 20 mins, turning once, halfway through.
3. Serve over chopped romaine lettuce with sliced avocado. Save any leftover chicken to use for lunch the next day.

Roasted shrimp and arugula chopped salad

Ingredients:

1 bunch of fresh asparagus spears (trimmed)

3 cups of arugula (roughly chopped)

1 lb of frozen shrimp (peeled and deveined, with tails intact)

1 cup of cherry tomatoes (halved)

½ of an avocado (peeled and sliced)

1 tbsp of pine nuts

4 tbsp of light, balsamic vinegar dressing

¼ of a tsp of salt

¼ of a tsp of pepper

Directions:

1. In a large skillet, pour a small amount of lightly-salted, boiling water over the asparagus, cover with a lid, and cook for 3 mins or until crisp-tender. Drain the asparagus in a colander and run under cold water until cool.

2. Place the asparagus on plates and top with the arugula, cooked shrimp, tomatoes, and avocado, and pine nuts. Drizzle with the light, balsamic vinegar dressing and sprinkle with salt and pepper to serve.

Flank steak with citrus marinade

Ingredients:

- 2 lbs of flank steak (or skirt steak)
- 1 orange (juiced)
- 1 lime (juiced)
- 4 garlic cloves (peeled and crushed)
- 2 tsp of brown mustard
- 1 ½ tbsp of apple cider vinegar

Directions:

1. Add the orange juice, lime juice, crushed garlic, mustard, and vinegar to a bowl and mix.
2. Place the steak in a resealable ziplock bag. Pour the marinade over the steak and refrigerate for 1–2 hours.
3. Preheat the grill to a medium–high heat And grill the steak for 6–7 mins per side, turning once.
4. Slice against the grain and serve with grilled asparagus or peppers.

Four-Step Method to Simple and Healthy Fish Dishes

A fish dish is an easy way to add some lean, healthy protein and crucial Omega fats to your diet. Simply choose a fish, some fresh herbs and seasonings, and some fresh produce from the lists below, and follow the grilling instructions.

Step 1 – Pick your fish

Try to choose wild-caught fish whenever possible; prepare 2 lbs of your selected fish:

- Salmon fillets
- Ahi tuna
- Mahi mahi
- Swordfish
- Snapper

Step 2 – Pick your herbs and seasonings

Roughly chop ½ of a cup of the following (except where noted):

- Basil
- Parsley
- Mint
- Dill
- Cilantro
- Chives
- Oregano
- Marjoram
- Garlic (3 cloves; minced)
- Ginger (½ in piece; peeled and grated)

Step 3 – Pick your fresh produce

Make use of some of the wonderful, seasonal produce available in stores and at farmer's markets:

- Heirloom tomatoes (thinly sliced)
- Zucchini ribbons
- Peppers (thinly sliced)
- Red or yellow onions (thinly sliced)
- Asparagus spears (trimmed)
- Summer squash (thinly sliced)
- Eggplant (thinly sliced)
- Lemon (thinly sliced)

Step 4 – Create, assemble, and grill

Follow the directions below to prepare your grilled fish creations. There are limitless possibilities for light, fresh, and healthy fish dishes.

1. Preheat the grill to a medium–high heat. In a bowl, mix together the herbs and seasonings of your choice with 1 tsp salt and 1–2 tbsp of olive oil. Use the back of a spoon or a food processor to create a fine paste.
2. Lightly oil a heavy piece of aluminum foil that is slightly larger than your fish fillet. Place the fish piece on it, skin side down (if there is skin), and spread the

herb mixture evenly over the fish. Then layer your thinly sliced produce of choice so that it covers the fish.

3. Sprinkle the fish with ½ of a tsp of salt and ¼ of a tsp of pepper. Transfer the fish, on the foil, to a preheated grill. Cook for about 10 mins, or until the fish flakes easily with a fork. Cooking times will vary slightly based on the type and thickness of your fish fillets.

4. Slide the fish off the foil and onto your serving platter. Serve with a fresh salad.

Additional Dinner Suggestions

Below you will find additional dinner suggestions so that you never run out of ideas. Do not forget about the soup recipes in the previous section; the vegetable dish recipes in the following section; or the salads in the lunch section which are just as delicious at dinner time.

- **Bacon wrapped chicken breast** with a spinach salad.
- **Grilled steak** with kale and avocado salad.
- **Grilled shrimp and zucchini** drizzled with coconut oil, sea salt, and paprika.
- **Baked cod** drizzled with coconut oil, sea salt, and paprika.
- **Omelet** – fill with whichever meat and vegetables are on hand.

- **Roasted chicken breasts with sweet potatoes** and a side of cooked quinoa.
- **Grilled fish** of choice with carrots and parsnips sautéed in coconut oil.
- **Steak and eggs** with a side of roasted sweet potatoes.
- **Baked salmon** with roasted beets and some steamed asparagus.
- **Grilled chicken sausage and zucchini** halves brushed with coconut oil.
- **Pan-fried pork chops** with sautéed onions and apples.
- **Roasted turkey breasts** with carrots and parsnips.
- **Green tacos** – mix 1lb of cooked ground chicken or lean beef and season with cumin; add fresh cilantro, avocado slices, tomato, and lime juice; and wrap in romaine leaves like a taco.
- **Grilled chicken breast and zucchini** – season with coconut oil, sea salt, and garlic salt; serve with asparagus.
- **Bunless burger** – grill 1 lb of grass-fed, organic beef, bison, or turkey burgers. Top with diced tomatoes and red onion; wrap in lettuce leaves if desired.
- **Flank steak** – grill 2 lbs of seasoned flank steak for about 5 mins on each side. Serve with baked sweet potato.

- **Baked cod with spinach** – top 4 oz of cod with 1 tbsp of lemon juice, sea salt, and ½ tsp coconut oil. Bake at 400 °F for 10–12 minutes until the fish flakes easily with a fork; serve with steamed spinach.
- **Baked salmon and asparagus** – top wild salmon with 1 tsp of coconut oil, ½ a tsp of garlic salt, and thinly sliced lemon. Bake at 400 °F for about 15 min; serve with steamed asparagus.
- **Honey lemon salmon** – preheat the broiler and season 1 ½ oz of salmon fillet with salt and pepper. Broil for 5 mins; drizzle with ½ of a tbsp of honey and ½ of a tsp of fresh lemon juice and broil for an additional 2–5 minutes.

VEGETABLE DISHES

Oven-roasted asparagus

Ingredients:

1 lb of asparagus (ends trimmed off)

2 tbsp of extra virgin olive oil

2 cups of grape tomatoes (halved)

3 tbsp of crumbled goat cheese (optional)

1 tsp of fresh garlic (minced)

2 tbsp of balsamic vinegar

1 tsp of salt

Directions:

1. Preheat the oven to 400 °F. Place the asparagus in a bowl and toss with 1 tbsp of olive oil and ½ of a tsp of salt. Place the asparagus in a single layer on a baking sheet. Place in the oven and roast for 8–10 mins, or until tender. Remove to a serving platter and cover with foil to keep warm while you are making the tomatoes.

2. Heat 1 tbsp of olive oil in a large skillet over a medium-high heat. Add the tomatoes and garlic and cook for 2–3 minutes. Add in the balsamic vinegar and cook for 2 more minutes. Season with salt.

3. Top the asparagus with the tomato mixture and crumble goat cheese on top.

4. 5-minute Swiss chard and kale saute with pine nuts

Ingredients:

4 cups of kale and Swiss chard leaves (stems removed and leaves torn into bite-sized pieces)

3 tbsp of grapeseed or olive oil

2 tsp of apple cider vinegar or champagne vinegar

½ of a tsp salt

¼ of a cup of pine nuts, sunflower seeds, or pepitas

Directions:

1. Heat the oil in a large saute pan; add the greens, and cook for about 2 mins.
2. Once the greens have started to shrink down and soften, add the vinegar and salt, and cook for another 2 mins.
3. Add pine nuts (or seeds) And cook for 1 more min. Serve warm.

Spaghetti squash with garlic oil

Ingredients:

1 spaghetti squash (halved and seeded)

½ of a cup of parmesan cheese

¼ of a tsp of Italian seasoning

¼ of a tsp of red pepper flakes

6 garlic cloves

½ of a cup olive oil

1 cup of water

¼ of a tsp of ground black pepper

1 tsp of sea salt

Directions:

1. Preheat the oven to 350 °F. Place squash halves, cut side down, in a rimmed baking sheet with water and

cover with foil. Bake for 50 mins, until the skin begins to look wrinkled and the squash is tender.

2. While the squash is in the oven, heat the olive oil in a small saucepan over a medium heat. Add the garlic, red pepper flakes, and Italian seasoning; cook until the garlic begins to lightly brown (be careful, it will burn fast). Add the water, sea salt, and pepper, and bring to a boil for 2 mins.

3. Shred the squash with a fork so that it looks like spaghetti strands. Toss with the garlic oil and sprinkle with parmesan to serve.

Green beans and tomatoes with lemon dressing

Ingredients:

1 lb of fresh green beans (trimmed)

1 cup of tomatoes (diced)

3 tbsp of lemon juice (or lime)

3 tbsp of olive oil

1 tsp of wine vinegar

½ of a tsp of salt

¼ of a teaspoon of pepper

1 tsp of chives (finely chopped)

1 cup of tomatoes (diced)

Directions:

1. Steam or cook the green beans until they are tender. Place in a bowl and top with tomatoes.
2. In a small bowl, whisk together the remaining ingredients and pour them over the hot green beans and tomatoes.

9

FATTY LIVER DIET PROTOCOL CHECKLIST AND FINAL ADVICE

Now that I have explained the Fatty Liver Diet Protocol in detail, it is time to put a plan into action. Included in the following pages are an action checklist based on what we have discussed throughout this book to keep you on track; a summary list of foods to avoid; and a final grocery list to remind you of the best foods to purchase during your weekly shopping trips.

The most important thing to remember is that you should introduce these lifestyle changes slowly, rather than trying to implement them all at once. Just by making a few small, but very effective, changes each week, you will be making big strides towards your new lifestyle. The long-term success of this plan is dependent on incorporating these changes a little at a time. Trying to change every aspect of your lifestyle in a single day will cause you to feel overwhelmed, make it more difficult to sustain, and will not allow you to figure out which aspects are having the desired effects, and which are not suited to you.

As you are putting this plan into action, remember that it took years for the damage to occur in your liver so you are not going to be able to heal it overnight. Be patient, put the work in, and you will begin to see results. The changes you make today begin with you. Your dedication to your own health will ultimately determine the level of your success.

Fatty Liver Diet Protocol Checklist

Use the following checklist as your guide to making the healthy lifestyle changes necessary to get your liver, your weight, and your energy back for good. To start with, try to complete one or two of the suggestions each day. As you grow more comfortable, increase the number of suggestions you are trying to meet until you can do just about everything on the checklist every single day without even thinking about it. Before you know it, these suggestions will become unconscious habits and you will be well on your way to feeling healthier than you have in years.

- Start the day with eight ounces of water mixed with the juice from half of a lemon
- Take a probiotic with breakfast to repopulate the gut with good quality bacteria
- Take a quality multivitamin to cover any nutrient deficiencies
- Take a combination of liver healing supplements

- Sip bone broth at least once throughout the day
- Avoid processed foods, refined sugars, refined flours, and alcohol
- Avoid gluten, grains, and as much dairy as possible
- Eat plenty of green and colorful organic vegetables from the approved grocery list
- Eat some fermented foods such as sauerkraut, kimchi, or fermented vegetables
- Eat at least two meals from the Fatty Liver Diet Protocol meal plan
- Drink at least eight glasses of filtered water throughout the day
- Do a HIIT workout
- Take a moment to focus on your breathing and evaluate your stress levels
- Do something just for you
- Get 8 hours of sleep

Additional Tips for Success to Heal Fatty Liver

1. Be patient

This will not be an overnight process. Every step you take to heal your liver is a step towards a lifetime of health, if you stay committed. You will recognize your progress when your symptoms and health issues begin to lessen, heal, and eventually disappear. These small victories will lead to larger victories and soon you will feel amazing!

2. Plan ahead

Careful planning can dramatically reduce stress and mental fatigue. Take fifteen minutes each night to plan out the next day; from your recipes and meals, to your grocery shopping and exercise. Planning ahead helps to keep you on the right track. Take time to prepare a few food items or even whole meals ahead of time if you know that the following day is going to be a busy one for you. It is easy to fall off the healthy meal wagon if you are struggling to find time to cook every day; it becomes too tempting to grab something quick and unhealthy.

3. Stop multitasking

Just because our Ipads can complete multiple activities at once, does not mean that we can. Too many goals and projects makes you feel overwhelmed and leads to lots of unfinished tasks. Stay focused on one item at a time to reduce stress and mental fatigue.

4. Schedule that HIIT workout

You only need to take part in a HIIT workout for 10–20 minutes to get the maximum liver healing benefits. Whether it is as soon as you wake up in the morning while the kids are still asleep, during your lunch break, or while you are watching your favorite television show at night, you should always be able to find a few minutes to squeeze in a quick and powerful workout. Do not let yourself make excuses for why you cannot find 10–20 minutes throughout the day to do this.

5. Take a brain break

Amidst the busyness of each day, it is easy to just keep going and going. However, a brain break allows us to slow down, regroup our thoughts, and get ready for the next task. By resting our minds we can help to reduce the stress on the rest of our body, including our liver.

6. Take time to get away

Finding 15 minutes of silence each day rests the mind and refuels the body. Ideally, taking 15 minutes for yourself between the hours of 1-3 pm will help you to refocus and recharge. This does not have to be a nap; simply sitting in silence and/or the dark will do. Be sure to control your thoughts and not let them run wild during this time – this is a mini getaway, not a working vacation.

7. Unwind before bed

It is not uncommon for us to pack as many activities into the day as possible. We rush here, rush there, and then collapse into bed without giving our minds time to settle. Spend 10–15 minutes before bed unwinding; turn the television off, shut down the computer and the cell phone; and sit down and relax. This is a great time to drink some warm bone broth to calm down the body and relax the mind.

8. Get some sleep

Nothing recharges the mind and body like 7–9 hours of sleep per night. Research has shown us that in order for us to function at our optimum level we need to be sleeping. 5–6 hours per night may seem like enough but it is not; our mind only recharges within the 7–9 hour range. Sleep may be the most underrated aspect of our health. Do not neglect getting good regular sleep if you want to heal your body and get your energy back.

Foods to Avoid to Heal the Liver

All Sources of Alcohol

- Beer
- Hard cider
- Liquor and spirits
- Liqueurs
- Wine

Sugary Drinks

- All types of sodas (both regular and diet)
- Energy drinks
- Fruit juice
- Sports drinks

Baked Goods and Refined Grains

- Bagels
- Biscuits
- Breakfast cereals
- Buns
- Cakes
- Cookies
- Corn
- Doughnuts
- Muffins
- Pasta
- Pastries
- Pies
- Pizza crust
- Rice
- White bread

Processed Foods and Foods High in Saturated Fats

- All fried foods
- Canned meat
- Canned soups
- Canned vegetables
- Chips
- Cooking spray that is not olive or coconut oil

- Crackers
- Cured meat
- Deli meats
- French fries
- Hot dogs
- Margarine
- Mayonnaise
- Pretzels
- Salad dressing
- Seed oils ("vegetable oils" such as Crisco, Canola, corn, and soybean oil)

Some of the items on the "avoid" list are allowed if they are made with healthy fats instead of unhealthy fats, so read the label carefully or make your own. For example, mayonnaise is made from eggs, oil, lemon juice, and salt; as long as you use oil made from healthy fats, you can still have mayonnaise!

Foods to Eat to Heal Your Liver

Keep this list on hand and bring it with you to the grocery store. Make sure you always include foods from every category as part of your weekly shopping.

Lean Meats and Eggs

- Beef (grass-fed if possible)
- Bison

- Chicken
- Eggs (free range is best
- Pork (chops or tenderloin)
- Turkey
- Turkey or chicken sausage

Vegetables

- Artichokes
- Arugula
- Asparagus
- Bell peppers
- Bok choy
- Broccoli
- Brussels sprouts
- Cabbage
- Carrots
- Cauliflower
- Chard
- Chives
- Collard greens
- Garlic
- Kale
- Leeks
- Mushrooms
- Mustard greens

- Napa cabbage
- Onions
- Peas
- Peppers
- Pumpkin
- Radicchio
- Romaine lettuce
- Spinach
- Squash
- Sweet potatoes
- Taro
- Turnips
- Watercress
- Yams

Fruits

- Avocados
- Blackberries
- Blueberries
- Grapefruit
- Kiwi
- Lemons
- Limes
- Melons
- Pomegranates
- Raspberries

- Strawberries

Healthy Monounsaturated Oil

- Avocado oil
- Coconut oil
- Olive oil

Healthy Nuts and Seeds

- Almonds
- Brazil nuts
- Flax seeds
- Hemp seeds
- Pecans
- Pistachios
- Pine nuts
- Pumpkins
- Sesame seeds
- Walnuts

Seafood

- Anchovies
- Cod
- Halibut
- Mackerel

- Mahi mahi
- Salmon
- Sardines
- Shellfish (shrimp and scallops)
- Snapper
- Trout
- Tuna
- White fish

Herbs

- Basil
- Cilantro
- Lavender
- Lemongrass
- Oregano
- Parsley
- Rosemary
- Spearmint
- Thyme

Beans

- Black beans
- Chickpeas
- Dried peas
- Hummus

- Lentils
- Navy beans
- White beans

Probiotic-Rich Foods

- Fermented vegetables
- Full fat Greek yogurt
- Kefir
- Kimchi
- Kombucha
- Miso
- Sauerkraut
- Yogurt (watch for added sugar)

Healthy Drinks

- Bone broth
- Green tea
- Kombucha
- Organic coffee
- Water

Supplements

- Artichoke leaf extract
- Choline

- Dandelion root
- Ginger
- Milk thistle
- Probiotics
- Vitamin E

LEAVE A 1-CLICK REVIEW!

Customer reviews

★★★★★ 5 out of 5

7 global ratings

5 star		100%
4 star		0%
3 star		0%
2 star		0%
1 star		0%

I would be incredibly thankful if you could take 60 seconds to write a brief review on Amazon, even if it's just a few sentences!

https://amzn.to/3v1FxyP

P.S. Including a picture (like of the cover or table of contents) really adds influence to your review if you have an extra minute to do that. Thanks in advance for your help!

REFERENCES

1. Liver: Anatomy and Functions. (n.d.). John Hopkins Medicine. Retrieved September 10, 2021, from https://www.hopkinsmedicine.org/health/conditions-and-diseases/liver-anatomy-and-functions

2. The Liver: Boundless Anatomy and Physiology. (n.d.). Lumen Learning. Retrieved September 10, 2021, from https://courses.lumenlearning.com/boundless-ap/chapter/the-liver/

3. Kubes, P. & Jenne, C. (2018, April 26). *Immune Responses in the Liver.* National Library of Medicine. https://pubmed.ncbi.nlm.nih.gov/29328785/

4. The Gallbladder. (n.d.). Lumen Learning. Retrieved May 26, 2021, from https://courses.lumenlearning.com/boundless-ap/chapter/the-gallbladder/

5. Christiansen, S. (n.d.). *The Anatomy of the Gallbladder.* Very Well Health. Retrieved May 26 2021, from https://www.verywellhealth.com/gallbladder-anatomy-4788045

6. Haelle, T. (2015, August 15). *10 Essential Facts About Your Gallbladder.* Everyday Health. https://www.everydayhealth.com/news/essential-facts-about-your-gallbladder/

7. *Cholecystectomy.* (n.d.). Mayo Clinic. Retrieved May 28, 2021, from https://www.mayoclinic.org/tests-procedures/cholecystectomy/about/pac-20384818

8. *Alcohol-Induced Liver Disease.* (n.d.). John Hopkins Medicine. Retrieved June 2, 2021, from https://www.hopkinsmedicine.org/health/conditions-and-diseases/alcoholinduced-liver-disease

9. *Non-Alcoholic Fatty Liver Disease (NAFLD).* (n.d.). American College of Gastroenterology. Retrieved June 2, 2021, from https://gi.org/topics/fatty-liver-disease-nafld/

10. Lee, D. (2019, December 26). *What is Drug Induced Liver Disease?* MedicineNet. https://www.medicinenet.com/drug_induced_liver_disease/article.htm

11. *Diagnosis of NAFLD & NASH.* (n.d.). National Institute of Diabetes and Digestive and Kidney Disease. Retrieved June 10, 2021, from https://www.niddk.nih.gov/health-information/liver-disease/nafld-nash/diagnosis

12. *The Progression of Liver Disease.* (n.d.–a). American Liver Foundation. Retrieved June 11, 2021, from https://www.google.com/url?q=https://liverfoundation.org/liver-awareness-month-fibrosis/&sa=D&source=editors&ust=1631308344181000&usg=AOvVaw0mlGkpCpxSiMWL8fOnsHHq

13. *The Progression Of Liver Disease.* (n.d.–b). American Liver Foundation. Retrieved June 11, 2021, from https://liverfoundation.org/for-patients/about-the-liver/diseases-of-the-liver/cirrhosis/#information-for-the-newly-diagnosed

14. *The Progression of Liver Disease.* (n.d.–c). American Liver Foundation. Retrieved June 11, 2021, from https://liverfoundation.org/for-patients/about-the-liver/diseases-of-the-liver/liver-cancer/

15. Paddock, C. (2016, February 25). *High Salt Diet May Harm Liver.* Medical News Today. https://www.medicalnewstoday.com/articles/307028

16. Moro, E. (2015, January 20). *The Rise of the Mediterranean Diet.* Alimentarium. https://www.alimentarium.org/en/story/rise-mediterranean-diet

17. *Definition and Potential Health Benefits of the Mediterranean Diet.* (2014, July 24). National Center for Biotechnology Information. https://www.ncbi.nlm.nih.gov/pmc/articles/PMC4222885/

18. Nagle, M. (2020, November 17). *Mediterranean Diet Shown to Lower Blood Pressure in Older Adults.* Medical Express. https://medicalxpress.com/news/2020-11-mediterranean-diet-blood-pressure-older.html

19. *Cancer and the Mediterranean Diet: A Review.* (2019, September 2). National Center for Biotechnology Information. https://www.ncbi.nlm.nih.gov/pmc/articles/PMC6770822/